"For too long, we have considered Jacques Lacan a theorist who confines himself to human subjects, even if he stresses their inhuman qualities. Finally, *Zoological Lacan* arrives to rescue Lacan from this misunderstanding, which he himself provoked. Teddy Duncan Jr.'s masterwork will force you to think differently about both the thought of Lacan and about how we theorize animality. Bringing Lacan's thought to bear on the question of the animal, *Zoological Lacan* marks a fundamental turning point in animal studies."

Todd McGowan, *Professor of English, University of Vermont, USA*

Zoological Lacan

Zoological Lacan examines the importance of Lacanian theory for understanding animals by situating them within Lacan's thought, relying on the occasional and fleeting (but surprisingly consistent) statements on animality throughout his work.

Teddy Duncan Jr. considers questions about animal subjectivity and the epistemological challenges that animals present, suggesting that a return to Lacan can resolve many of the lacunas within our comprehension of them. Using the Lacanian triad (the symbolic, the imaginary, and the Real), Duncan develops a "Zoological Lacanianism" that not only delineates a psychoanalytic understanding of animal interiority but also supplies fresh insights into animal behavior and subjectivity, exceeding Lacan's direct comments on animality. This book extends Lacan's thought by providing new theoretical interventions on topics such as animal interiority, communication, guilt, jouissance, trauma, the unconscious, and human-animal love. While carefully avoiding collapsing the subjectivity of animals and humans, animals are shown to be psychoanalytic subjects. The book also reflects on the significance these areas can have for other fields such as philosophy, psychoanalysis, and animal studies.

Zoological Lacan announces—to the study of animals, psychoanalysis, and philosophy—that a new theory has emerged on the scene, one that warrants substantive and sustained engagement.

Teddy Duncan Jr. is an Associate Professor at Valencia College. His writing on psychoanalysis, literature, and animality has been published in various academic journals, and this is his second book.

The Lines of the Symbolic in Psychoanalysis Series

Series Editor: Ian Parker
Manchester Psychoanalytic Matrix

Psychoanalytic clinical and theoretical work is always embedded in specific linguistic and cultural contexts and carries their traces, traces which this series attends to in its focus on multiple contradictory and antagonistic 'lines of the Symbolic'. This series takes its cue from Lacan's psychoanalytic work on three registers of human experience, the Symbolic, the Imaginary and the Real, and employs this distinctive understanding of cultural, communication and embodiment to link with other traditions of cultural, clinical and theoretical practice beyond the Lacanian symbolic universe. The Lines of the Symbolic in Psychoanalysis Series provides a reflexive reworking of theoretical and practical issues, translating psychoanalytic writing from different contexts, grounding that work in the specific histories and politics that provide the conditions of possibility for its descriptions and interventions to function. The series makes connections between different cultural and disciplinary sites in which psychoanalysis operates, questioning the idea that there could be one single correct reading and application of Lacan. Its authors trace their own path, their own line through the Symbolic, situating psychoanalysis in relation to debates which intersect with Lacanian work, explicating it, extending it and challenging it.

Writings for a Liberation Psychoanalysis
Politicizing the Unconscious from the Core of a Crumbling Empire
Robert K. Beshara

Psychoanalysing Mind-Body Narratives Through Beckett and Artaud
The Trauma of the Body
Sarah Meehan O'Callaghan

Zoological Lacan
A Lacanian Framework for Animality
Teddy Duncan Jr.

For more information about the series, please visit: https://www.routledge.com/The-Lines-of-the-Symbolic-in-Psychoanalysis-Series/book-series/KARNLOS

Zoological Lacan

A Lacanian Framework for Animality

Teddy Duncan Jr.

Routledge
Taylor & Francis Group
LONDON AND NEW YORK

Designed cover image: Getty Images

First published 2027
by Routledge
4 Park Square, Milton Park, Abingdon, Oxon OX14 4RN

and by Routledge
605 Third Avenue, New York, NY 10158

Routledge is an imprint of the Taylor & Francis Group, an informa business

British Library Cataloguing-in-Publication Data
A catalogue record for this book is available from the British Library

ISBN: 978-1-041-06431-2 (hbk)
ISBN: 978-1-041-06430-5 (pbk)
ISBN: 978-1-003-63538-3 (ebk)

DOI: 10.4324/9781003635383

Typeset in Times New Roman
by Apex CoVantage, LLC

For Papa

Contents

Acknowledgments

From one vantage, a book is a temporal investment—the author dedicates time to an idea (or a cluster of interrelated ideas, organized by some central concept) for a prolonged period, eventually (hopefully) culminating in publication. We all have a finite amount of time at our disposal (and somehow this finitude seems more apparent today, despite the putatively increasing conveniences of contemporary life), and writing a book certainly reminds one of that fact. Acknowledgements recognize, however, that not only the author's time has been invested—and I acknowledge the following people for giving up their attention and time for me and this project in different ways.

I thank everyone at Routledge for their willingness and enthusiasm for taking on this project, in particular, Susannah Frearson, Eleanor Taylor, and Saloni Singhania. I would also like to thank Ian Parker, the editor of the "Lines of the Symbolic" series, for giving me the opportunity to situate my work among some of the best Lacanian scholarship—I am extremely proud to be part of this series. I also deeply appreciate the anonymous peer reviewers for their substantive and astute feedback that undoubtedly improved the manuscript.

Beyond peer reviewers and those at Routledge, I also thank everyone who looked over sections of the manuscript and provided feedback: Bruce Janz, Rudy McDaniel, and Jonathan Beever. Their feedback ensured that my work had something to say beyond the Lacanians among us—thank you for your encouraging commentary. I also thank Todd McGowan for his endorsement of the book: his comments confirmed, to me, that I was handling this territory properly and making a worthwhile contribution.

The theory reading group in Tampa, begun by John Lennon, was imperative for the formation of these ideas: the group provided a space to articulate my thoughts to those much smarter than myself (and gave me deeper insights into both Freudian and Kleinian theory). Thank you for letting me listen to your incisive thoughts on texts each month: John Lennon, Maria Cizmic, Andrew Berish, Meg Hanna, April Young, Ben Fried, and Olivia Cosentino. John Lennon was indispensable to this project. Though our theoretical and scholarly territory has diverged, his insight into the publication process and support for my work is largely the reason I have been able to navigate the world of academic publishing with any degree of confidence. I hope one day to have the same impact on one of my students as he has had on me.

Additionally, thank you to my friends at UCF who have supported my work, in particular: Christina, Erin, Glenn, LJ, and Tyler.

Thank you to my students at Valencia College—despite being a corny platitude, it is true that you learn more from teaching than one could ever teach. Also, thank you to my colleagues at Valencia, particularly Doug Kern, who is an extraordinary collaborator and friend.

My friends, who once again, when I wasn't in monk mode working on this project, provided much-needed relief through skating or hiking or talking—Carlos, Dert, Elias, Eliseo, Guzman, Jon, Luis, Mendez, Seth, Simon, and Quinn. Thank you all.

Thank you to my cat, Cashmere. (I hope you're okay with the preface.)

My family (who all compassionately nodded their heads in agreement as I tried, unsuccessfully, to describe my next book project) are the reason this text exists. I'd do anything to make you all proud. Thank you to my mother, father, Nana, aunts, uncles, cousins—as well as Rosaura and Nhuyen. Without your love and support, I wouldn't get beyond the first page.

Zena, thank you for your love and patience, once again. I'm sorry for the books littering the living room and for putting off washing the dishes until I got to the end of a sentence. I love and adore you.

Finally, I dedicate this book to my grandfather, Marion Duncan—Papa's love for his family was inexhaustible, and I hope to be a fragment of who he was.

Series Preface

One of the fundamental underlying shifts in our conception of ourselves as human beings that psychoanalysis forces us to confront is that we are de-centred, inhuman. Freud argued this point quite explicitly, and Lacan insisted upon it. Just as Copernicus showed us that our little planet is not the centre of the universe, and Darwin showed us that the human being is not the pinnacle of creation, so psychoanalysis shows us that we are not the masters in the house. Humanist nostrums disintegrate along with the hope that we could become the very sun around which we ourselves revolve.

We are, rather, implicated in the lives of others, and in every form of life which we so often take such pains to distinguish ourselves from, unable now to even conceptualise ourselves as strutting on the earth as if it were a stage—a well-meaning image of our place here that underpins much environmental discourse—coming face to face with our imbrication in that environment and its many kinds of beings, and with arguments that go beyond environmentalism to ecology. Our inhumanity is then not redeemed by psychoanalysis, but questioned, and this book on animality in psychoanalysis—a zoological return to Lacan—refuses to take refuge in moral claims, staying with that ethical puzzling that brings us the closest to what it is to be a sentient being.

This extraordinary book attends to the three dimensions Lacan mapped, of the symbolic, the imaginary and the real, tracing its way through domains that we think are familiar, but defamiliarizing each of them in an investigation of the openings, consequences and traps that Lacan himself sets as we venture into his territory, into his own return to Freud. This requires elaboration of what it means to distinguish the sign from the signifier, and how it is possible to situate ourselves and the animals we encounter and symbolise and fantasise about. It requires that we notice, again anew, how we are captured by the imaginary we evoke when we declare that it is animals void of the signifier who are captured by that imaginary register. And it requires that we encounter a real that is, as if, abolished at the moment that the animals, ourselves included, are named, when our word is the murder of the thing.

Psychoanalytic clinical and theoretical work circulates through multiple intersecting antagonistic symbolic universes. This series opens connections between different cultural sites in which Lacanian work has developed in distinctive ways, in forms of work that question the idea that there could be a single correct reading and application. The Lines of the Symbolic in Psychoanalysis series provides a reflexive reworking of psychoanalysis that transmits Lacanian writing from around the world, steering a course between the temptations of a metalanguage and imaginary reduction, between the claim to provide a god's eye view of psychoanalysis and the idea that psychoanalysis must everywhere be the same. And the elaboration of psychoanalysis in the symbolic here grounds its theory and practice in the history and politics of the work in a variety of interventions that touch the real.

Ian Parker
Manchester Psychoanalytic Matrix

Preface: A Complicated Subject (The Cat Who Bites My Legs)

The unpredictable, fluid proclivities of a cat patently render them a complicated subject, and by 'subject' I do not merely reduce cats to the register of scientism (as in the 'subject' of study that is, in reality, viewed as an object—the empirically quantifiable subject-object with no view of its own) but as an experiential 'subject,' meaning an agent equipped with implacable (and undeniable) interiority, who perceives and is aware of that which is perceived, introducing a horizon of subjectivity and life; a subject who approaches the world, however uncertainly, however tentatively, however eloquently or ineloquently and, guided by some internal mechanism (whether this self-governing apparatus consists of pre-dispositions, instincts, or freewill is not pertinent, at this juncture, in defining them as an authentic 'subject'), self-elects (to some degree or another) what is to be done within that encountered world. A cat, for anyone who has ever observed one, is indisputably a subject in the latter sense as much as anyone (or anything) can be a subject (meaning object) in the former sense. By this I mean cats are a subject of experience, albeit complicated ones. Jacques Derrida, in his posthumously published book *The Animal That Therefore I Am*, observes that a confrontation—an exchange of gaze—with a cat reminds us of their "unsubstitutable singularity,"[1] prompting a crisis of humanness. A cat, in all their unresolvable complexity (which cannot be settled by being 'subjected' to an analysis on the plane of species), demands to be contended with on the individuated level.

As Derrida says, when one really encounters a cat, they are not encountering a "figure of a cat . . . an allegory for all the cats on the earth" but a "real cat"[2]—one that "looks at me . . . she and no other."[3] Yet, clearly, the cat which Derrida encounters is not entirely available to his gaze—the encounter with the cat leaves a remainder that is unassimilable; there is some interiority to the cat (the cat who stares, not to be conflated with archetypal cathood itself) that defies the calculating gaze of human knowledge. A cat remains, in some sense, unavailable and concealed by an opaque screen of subjectivity. As Jacques Lacan writes, "speaking of the subject . . . presents us with a sort of unknowable substance, something resistant to objectification."[4] This is why confronting the animal as a subject rather than an object is a radical gesture—because it recognizes the "unknowable substance" central to being.

In her book *Sexual Personae*, Camille Paglia also detects the latent impenetrability of cats as subjects:

> Cats have secret thoughts, a divided consciousness. No other animal is capable of ambivalence, those ambiguous cross-currents of feeling, as when a purring cat simultaneously buries its teeth warningly in one's arm.[5]

We see here that, according to Paglia's observations, a cat is not merely a transparent subjected-subject that we enact indubitable control over or even maintain precise, objective knowledge of—a cat is a subject which remains hidden behind ambivalent inscrutability. The cat presents the limit of human knowledge: A living, ineffable being that can both purr and bite and leave the interpretative division between the two (attachment and aggression; love and hate) for the human to decipher. A cat is an-other in the same sense in which any human we encounter is an-other: the one who-is-not-us is always a site of alterity (and, according to psychoanalysis, we are even an-other to ourselves because of the Other—the unconscious, issuing from inside us, is a point of self-alterity). While it may be excessive for Paglia to solely confer this mode of ambivalence to cats (and thereby definitionally exclude all other animals from this capacity), it is unequivocally, even empirically, true that cats are culturally representative of this ambivalent impenetrability. Cats are subjects who are, in a word, complicated. If animals are normally presumed to be simpler creatures—as creatures who are thrusted forward by nothing more than the life-drive, the Freudian pleasure-principle, and, if they are granted a subjectivity at all, this subjectivity is presupposed to operate according to simple evolutionary mechanisms—then cats, as an illustrative counter-example, compel us to re-consider the interiority of animals.

Like Derrida, when I encounter the cat in the hallway, I am presented with a partially opaque, inscrutable subject that eludes the reductive register of scientism: There is something more (complicated) in the cat than a subject oriented purely by a life-drive. A cat (this cat, the actual, non-figurative, non-representational one I gaze at in the hallway, named Cashmere with orange fur and stripe-like wisps of dark-orange on the cusp of brown) is not bound to the binarized biological processes of attachment and aggression, joy and fear. The cat-subject lies on her back and purrs, offering her belly and inviting a pet—and when I extend my arm, reaching towards her belly-fur, she deftly attacks me with the same playful ambivalence that Paglia describes; she sinks her teeth slowly into the side of my hand (with perceptible joy and subtle, ambivalent, love-aggression). In the morning, as I walk to the kitchen in shorts, she bites my bare legs and aggressively meows, scratching at the closet door concealing her kibble food, deploying communicative gestures demanding I feed her. I pour the food in her bowl, walk away, and she promptly bites my leg again, runs away (with glee?) and furtively hides beneath a chair. She refuses to be placed anywhere; she prefers to situate herself. I place her on the couch beside me, and she leaps off. At times, she jumps on my desk (the one place I would prefer her not to leap onto), perches on her hind legs, and incomprehensibly stares at my face—an inaccessible, inexhaustible gaze—and brushes against my hand, asking in a corporeal-gestural language to be pet. I pet her face; she bites my fingers. She meows at doors in a high and insistent pitch, begging them to be opened, then walks into the doorway of a newly accessible room—and departs back through the same doorway seconds later. At night, she curls at my feet and attentively claws my toes. She vocalizes; she desires; she chooses; she expresses.

Cashmere is not totally unknowable—sometimes, fleetingly, she appears utterly transparent; her usual opacity is shed by a communicative transmission. Her pain, for example, is marked by explicit external signs: She howls and hides, even refusing food if the pain reaches a certain unbearable threshold. She has preferences that cannot be denied, though those preferences are liable to sudden change. She prefers the space on the carpet in the living room where sunlight escapes through the blinds. Other times, she prefers the darkness beneath the bed. Totalizing, complete access may not be possible (I cannot feel her pain—I cannot know why her preferences shift over time from the couch to beneath the bed to the patch of sunlight on the carpet), but she is a subject that can be known. Cashmere can be known while remaining, in the final interpretation, unknowable. Her ambivalence is unresolvable, intractable—I know when she vocalizes in the morning—*meow meowww meow*—she demands food, but I do not know why she bites my leg after I feed her.

Why does the cat bite my leg? We could reductively categorize the ambivalence of the bite as 'play'—she is only playing, and playing is the very enactment of non-serious aggression, enabled by the pretense of pretend (if one can decisively ascribe to a cat the capacity of pretense, that is). Simply, it is the emission of violence through means that are actually, in their intentionality, non-violent. Yet, there is a lingering sense of authentic emotiveness (leaks of a complicated subjectivity): At times, there is disdain (the bite that denotes excessive petting has taken place—non-verbally informing me, *that's enough!*) and at other times, there is pure affection (the rub of the head against my hand; the clawed paw placed softly, with care, on my face). The cat (the real cat who bites, gazes, and defecates) cannot be tabulated through an ethological-economical analysis that interpretatively informs us of every action's meaning; the cat who bites my legs exceeds this analysis and remains partly epistemically impenetrable.

A cat may appear, at times, ambivalent and inscrutable, but what of those animals more capable of a direct, unmistakable self-disclosure, such as those who employ sign-language in place of speech-acts and even participate, at the margins, in what we would likely call 'human' activity? Specifically, how should primates be situated in the field of animality and its putative ambivalences? One primate, named Travis, lived with a family for one-and-a-half decades in Connecticut, and his preferences and sufferings appear transparent enough:

> Sandy and Jerry invited Travis to join them at the table for meals. He ate oatmeal with a spoon every morning. At their favorite Italian restaurant, Pellicci's, she read him the menu, offering him choices. His favorite food was filet mignon. He also enjoyed lobster tail. He preferred Lindt's chocolates. He liked Nerds

> candy and taffy, and he loved ice cream, hooting and pulling at Sandy when the ice-cream man came down the street. When he was thirsty, he swung his body up onto the counter and took out a glass, opened the refrigerator, and poured himself juice or soda.[6]

Travis's subjectivity was not unavailable to those around him: socially, he was knowable. He dined at a table and slept in a bed and rode in cars and, by all signs, loved. In 1999, he mauled a family friend's face, nearly killing her, right outside the suburban home he was raised in. Aside from some disturbances earlier that day—slightly erratic behavior—amounting to low-level annoyance by his adopted 'mother,' there was no identifiable causal event that preceded the mauling. Travis had met this woman many times before and exhibited no aggressive behavior. This anecdote should remind us of the mystery of animal thought. However, we are also disturbed by the sudden murder-suicide in the middle-class neighborhood (perpetrated by the language-speaking and tax-paying human), searching in vain for a sufficient explanatory reason for the act. The mystery of the animal is merely the mystery of the other compounded.

"Startle," the opening poem of Kate Sweeney's *Worrisome Creatures*, chronicles a commonplace event that dramatizes, in a revealing way, this mode of encounter with the animal other. In this case, it is an encounter with a deer in the early morning. After seeing the deer, she writes, "the first sun waits/to burn through/and expose us all/standing on spindle legs/eye's wet/waiting for the other to spook."[7] In these lines, we should note that it is not just the deer "standing on spindle legs"—it is us as well. We are similarly 'exposed.' The deer and the human occupy the same position in relation to each other—a position of fear and apprehension—they are both 'startled' or 'spooked' by the other. Us and the deer, on our 'spindle legs,' are locked in an encounter, a deadlock—and this truly is a substantive 'event.' But why does the deer spook us? And why do we spook the deer? It is the other's inaccessibility that is 'startling'—an encounter 'spooks' us because we do not have direct access to another. Like Derrida, Paglia, and myself, Sweeney catalogues the glimpse of an animal's impenetrable specificity: An animal's eyes—the animal gaze—conceals a subjectivity that does not freely offer itself up to the human gaze. When encountering the human gaze, we surmise what we can: we tell ourselves (falsely), *I could tell by his look what he was thinking*, and the subject can confirm or deny this intuition through language—yet when confronting the animal gaze we perceive an entirely full blankness; a blankness that does not indicate emptiness but a hidden horizon of subjectivity in absence of the normal self-revealing emissions available to humans, namely the faulty self-assuredness of language. An encounter with animals prompts the question, asked by the psychoanalyst André Green about drives, "How may language gain access to the language of what lies beyond language?"[8] To which we must re-articulate as: How may language gain access to the language of what lies beyond language, namely the animal?

When contending with the subjectivity of another human, we rely on the symbolic universe for access to their interiority. We ask each other: What are you thinking about? Despite the potential dubiousness of the response (due to the inexorable severance between signification and 'true thought'—the alienating operation of language) or the prospect of a misapprehension between transmission (due to the constitutive misalignment of signifiers) or even intent to deceive by the other (due to the other's desire to manipulate or conceal), we often take that response as a genuine representation of one's subjective condition. For animals, we have no such recourse to language—but this does not mean they must be cast as forever unknowable. We could consider the cat's tail as a site offering partial knowability: informing us when they are angry, frustrated, or scared. The tail does not offer the ostensible assuredness of language, where one supplies self-commentary on their own experience intersubjectively communicated to an-other, but the tail does intimate the structure of an animal-subject's interiority. This is a basic insight that we are all—to one degree or another—aware of.

This is the precise entry-point that my book begins at: Not with the asinine insight that animals are transparently available by ethological or psychological research (that animals are reducible to economic-machines of instinct) nor that animals must remain a totally impenetrable mystery-void (that knowledge of animals is unattainable and only subject to speculative conjecture)—animals are subjects that are neither epistemically impossible nor auto-available (and hence not empty of interiority). Animals are subjects that are complicated, but a complicated status does not preclude them from a scrupulous and illuminative analysis ('complicated' does not denote the impossibility of a disclosure of subjectivity)—and, as I will explicate in the ensuing pages, no other thinker than Jacques Lacan offers a more apt framework for detailing this abyss of animal subjectivity. Through Lacanian theory, both the animal subject and the human subject enter a more refined mode of analysis and subsequently re-emerge in greater epistemic focus—the abyss that animal interiority presents can be lessened, though in no way am I claiming the chasm will ever be totally overcome.

Notes

1 Jacques Derrida, *The Animal That Therefore I Am*, ed. Marie-Louise Mallet, trans. David Wills (New York: Fordham University Press, 2008), 9.
2 Derrida, *The Animal That Therefore I Am*, 8.
3 Derrida, *The Animal That Therefore I Am*, 9.
4 Jacques Lacan, *The Formations of the Unconscious: The Seminar of Jacques Lacan*, Book V, ed. Jacques-Alain Miller, trans. Russell Grigg (Cambridge: Polity Press, 2017), 93.
5 Camille Paglia, *Sexual Personae: Art and Decadence from Nefertiti to Emily Dickinson* (New Haven: Yale University Press, 1990), 66.
6 Dan Lee, "Travis the Menace," *New York Magazine*, 2011.
7 Kate Sweeney, *Worrisome Creatures* (Dallas, TX: Madville Publishing, 2022), 1.
8 André Green, *On the Destruction and Death Drives*, trans. Steven Jaron, ed. Howard B. Levine (London: Phoenix Publishing House, 2023), 98.

Introduction

Zoological Lacanianism

Jacques Lacan announced in 1953—when introducing his famous paper "The Function and Field of Speech and Language in Psychoanalysis," in which he explicitly heralded his signifier-centric mode of theory—that psychoanalysis, post-Freud, had atrophied into a "technique . . . one that is gloomy in style" and it now tacitly prohibited "any attempt to let in critical fresh air."[1] An intellectual attrition of the psychoanalytic project had taken place; Freud's idiosyncratic approach (drawing from literature, art, personal anecdote, and the sciences) had been supplanted by a restrictive dogma in the name of scientific legitimacy. Lacan, in his statement, was effectively declaring his own critical intervention in psychoanalysis and injection of "critical fresh air," through his already-begun 'return to Freud,' eventually solidifying into its own iteration of psychoanalytic thought bearing his name.

Lacan's 'return to Freud' was a pivotal theoretical move—not only was Lacan's move one that re-designated Freudianism as more than just the historical-conceptual foundation of psychoanalysis, but Lacan also envisioned the future of psychoanalysis as predicated on a non-regressive excavation of Freud's texts and ideas. Freud's work, for Lacan, was not merely the past originary material of the psychoanalytic discourse; it was instead meant to function as the mediator for where that discourse should continue on to. While others viewed Freudianism as functionally archaic and fully exhausted against the emergence of new empirical-positivist research and psychological theories, or were taking psychoanalysis in new directions by deliberately neglecting certain Freudian ideas, Lacan maintained that the true insights of Freud had not been properly contended with by the psychoanalytical world—there were paths, before he intervened, that remained unexhausted and partially undiscovered. Freud had written extensively on psychoanalytic theory and practice—causing a Copernican revolution of our understanding of interiority—but according to Lacan, the full implications and meaning of Freudian theory had yet to be uncovered.

However, we should not delude ourselves: Lacan's return to Freud was not a true 'return' in the sense of having absolute fidelity to the source—Lacan's Freud was not Freud's own Freud, but a Freud interpreted through the prism of Lacan's (supra-structuralist and later Real/jouissance-oriented) project. This is where Lacan's assertion is truly radical: by taking Freud's texts and channeling them through

DOI: 10.4324/9781003635383-1

his own ideas, Lacan retroactively generated the Freud to which he was to return. In a sense, Lacan discovered the 'true' Freud by extrapolating concepts from his theories that Freud himself never considered. There was a distinctly hermeneutical element to this discovery—it was a particular reading of Freud which, paradoxically, without distortion, led him to the place of Freudian truth. And, while it is incontestable this is not the same truth that Freud himself (or, at least the textual Freud we engage with by reading his work or the biographical Freud of historicity we will never know) subscribed to, it is equally unequivocal that Lacan's Freud is indeed textually and theoretically present in his work—he did not place something entirely alien to the Freudian field and manage to somehow derive insights incompatible with Freud's approach.

Lacan goes so far as to admit this play with Freudian doctrine and his texts, stating in *The Ethics of Psychoanalysis* that "on occasion I know how to take liberties with Freud's texts and affirm my distance."[2] It is apparent, for an astute reader of Freud and Lacan, that Lacanian theory at times holds a certain "distance" from the Freudian source, taking occasional "liberties" with the material. Lacan subsequently, in that same passage, describes the "dominance" of the signifier as an example of his deviation from strict Freudian doctrine—yet, at times, he defends the emphasis on signifiers as already-present in Freud's work. Always reminding his audience that, while it may not (cannot) be explicitly present in Freud's work, the theory of the signifier is implicitly present, even preceding the discovery in linguistics by Ferdinand De Saussure of the signifier/signified binary and its 'structural' function. Lacan claims, unequivocally, that Freud "brings out a dimension that no one had ever suggested before him. This dimension is precisely that of the signifier."[3] (Though Freud certainly never referred to the signifier as such.)

One must consider the true operation of Lacan's return to Freud: he is returning to Freud by returning to that which never existed. In a real sense, though, it now exists—and, of course, this is what we now refer to as Lacanian thought. It is clear why this move perturbed so many in the psychoanalytic community and led to so many personal and professional issues for Lacan (such as his 'excommunication' from the international body of psychoanalysis, the International Psychoanalytic Association): Lacan was effectively a heretic. If Freud is the Godhead of psychoanalysis, Lacan's entrance was marked by an arrogant, blasphemous declaration: *I have found exactly what God himself could not see.* Note that this heretical declaration does not assert that God is wrong; but, rather, that God is limited (or, that the original apostles were deficient in their early interpretations, lacking the necessary revelatory perceptiveness to understand God's message) and that only through the heretic's interpretation (which infuses new meaning into the text but does not exactly exceed its conceptual bounds) could God be apprehended. In the theology of psychoanalysis, while he defers to God (Freud), Lacan also establishes himself as the one true Prophet—and this Prophet, like all his predecessors, divulged his own revelations to the (clinical) clergy, as well as the (non-clinical) laity.

Undoubtedly, Lacan led to psychoanalysis letting in 'critical fresh air' between the mid-20th century and today (the proliferation of books on Lacan in disparate fields and disciplines is evidence of this fact). However, since Lacan's death in 1981, psychoanalysis (especially the Freudo-Lacanian strain) has been in conspicuous worldwide decline, often dismissed as an artifact from the 20th century that is excavated for its political, philosophical, or literary insights (particularly in the United States), and relegated to humanities departments as 'theory.' The designation as 'theory' is not, inherently, a negative appellation—but the academy seems to have forgotten that Lacan's theories, since they emerged from the clinical domain, have applications beyond texts and philosophy. Circumscribing Lacanian theory to conventional literary texts and cultural studies is precisely the reason it has maintained a peculiar omission on one subject: Animality.

With Lacan, and particularly his treatment within the study of animality, there is a similar history—animal theorists and scientists feel that they have effectively 'moved past' Lacan and his theories. There is a 'gloominess' and a reluctance to permit 'fresh air' in on the animal question. Theorists believe that they had successfully transcended the limits of his theoretical views, that he effectively has nothing to offer. Those in the 'hard sciences' neglect his work as un-rigorous and non-empirical, and those in the animal studies-adjacent 'humanities' feel Lacan's work has little, if anything, to offer our understanding of animals. Gautam Basu Thakur and Jonathon Michael Dickstein, in their introduction to the edited collection *Lacan and the Nonhuman*, write that critics suggest "Freudian-Lacanian psychoanalysis is simply incompatible with the non-human turn."[4] Chapters later, Kevin Andrew Spicer explains why this is the case:

> There has been no small quantity of ink spilled showing that Lacan's work will not really help one talk about the nonhuman at all. His thought is just another exemplary case of "structural linguistic correlationism" ([Adrian] Johnston); a typical anthropocentric humanist who cannot think the nature of the animal ([Jacques] Derrida); or perhaps worst of all, a scatological thinker whose worry about what humans will do with their "shit" keeps him from articulating the "ecological thought" so necessary to today in the Anthropocene ([Timothy] Morton).[5]

Even in *Lacan and the Nonhuman*, which is the sole book on Lacanian thought that takes into account the non-human or animal turn and argues convincingly throughout for the application of Lacanian thought in this field, few of the authors use Lacan to understand animal interiority.

Like Lacan recognized in Freud, I see that Lacanian thought has not been properly contended with—that we have not exhausted Lacan; we have, instead, looked past him for the very insights which his texts can provide. I propose, as Lacan himself did in 1953, a return to a theoretical model which has, for certain reasons, gone out of fashion: We need a return to Lacan (in a field which has not yet embraced his theories). However, I acknowledge that, in a sense, this is a return to that which-has-not-yet-existed. I do not wish to distort Lacan; rather, I seek to give Lacan a proper articulation in a new field—the field of animal studies.

When Lacan initiated his return to Freud, he always emphasized how this return acted upon a foundation left by Freud's own writings. Lacan writes in Seminar V, discussing Freud's account of witticism and the unconscious:

> What point would there be in talking about Freud if we didn't try to derive the maximum benefit from what he contributed? It's up to us to move it along a little further by giving it this formalization, and our experience will tell us whether it is right and whether this is the right direction for organizing the phenomena.[6]

We see here the exact appeal I am making: An attempt to "move it [psychoanalytic theory] along a little further" through "formalization" of something that is otherwise incompletely formulated. Unlike Lacan's return to Freud, however, I *recognize* that I am not a prophet: this is not the Lacan that Lacan himself may have deliberately developed, but, concurrently, this is no distortion: the insights are textually present within his work, and the derivative implications I will present for animals are unequivocally Lacanian (without being Lacan's own). Calling this Lacanian or Post-Lacanian is not a substantive distinction—it is a return to Lacan in the lineage of Lacan's return to Freud.

This should not be an unexpected development, though it may be not intentionally pre-explicated in his work: like Lacan's introduction of structuralist linguistics to Freud's thought (which was unanticipated by the historical figure Freud, but prefigured in his works such as *Interpretations of Dreams*, *The Psychopathology of Everyday Life*, and *Jokes and Their Relation to the Unconscious*); Lacan did not intend to produce a coherent theory of animality, and surely could not anticipate the prominence of the 'animal turn.' However, throughout his writings, there are glimpses of a semi-systematic line of thought on animal interiority. Consolidating these fragments of Lacan's work into an organized theoretical system generates a return to that which does not exist—a Lacanian theory of animality. Katie Gentile argues in her article "Animals as *the* Symptom of Psychoanalysis" that animality is pervasively embedded in psychoanalytic theory, all the way from the progenitor, Freud himself. Gentile perceptively (and correctly) writes,

> the animal is always present as the symptom, the Id, the primitive ego, the drive, the libido, the instinct, the body. The animal *is* the unspoken and implicit focus of psychoanalytic exploration and engagement to organize, tame, and harness the animal.[7]

We see this, of course, in the famous case studies of Freud, such as the 'Rat-Man' and 'Wolf-Man' and Little Han's horse-phobia—where an animal is representationally tethered to the symptom.

The animal is present from the very origins of psychoanalysis, but animality in its authentic non-human alterity is rarely contended with; instead, "psychoanalysis emerges only *with* a particular intimacy with animals," and this has led to very "little written directly about animals within psychoanalysis."[8] Animals are representatively present in psychoanalysis, as proxy-figures of unconscious desires, but the psychoanalytic implications of the animal themselves are not taken into account—and, as Gentile observes, when psychoanalysts do theorize animality, "they did so with headache-inducing contradictions and ambivalences."[9] Although Gentile never mentions Lacan in her article, he perfectly corresponds to this characterization: There are certainly, at times, irreconcilable contradictions in his writings on animality, using the animal to define the human, and merely relying on the animal as a representation of human desires. However, we also find in Lacan's seminars and *Écrits* a willingness to approach the abyss of animality and not merely reduce it to the not-quite-human; Lacan supplies us with profound insights, sometimes tentatively and mostly digressively, on animality. Lacan's resistance to privileging the ego and his unique conception of the 'subject,' both imperative to his psychoanalytic project, permit this unique confrontation with animality.

We must not follow the delusory approach which extracts material from Lacan's work and neglects its purpose. Although Lacan's writings and seminars have indelibly altered the stream of distinct academic disciplines, he clearly states on multiple occasions that, "[t]he goal of my teaching has always been, and remains, to train analysts."[10] The essential kernel of his writings and thought remains bound to this goal. As Charles Shepardson writes, Lacan's interactions and references to other disciplines, such as philosophy, should not be mis-apprehended as functioning within that discourse, since he is pursuing psychoanalytic truths "mobilized in the interest of the clinical domain."[11] Regardless, Lacan opens up new spaces within those discursive domains which he interacts with for the sake of psychoanalysis: animal studies must properly situate and integrate the Lacanian insights without reducing him to a pure philosopher or literary theorist. Simply—there is no such thing as Lacanian thought outside of the psychoanalytic ground in which his ideas were dedicated to and emerged from; one cannot successfully sever Lacan from the conceptual circumstances that underlie his writings. Lacan is a psychoanalyst whose insights are irreducible to psychoanalysis.

To a Place That Does Not Exist . . .

Lacan, in his own writings and seminars, unbarred the theoretical aperture I am attempting to pass through (I am not, myself, the one who established the place of the animal in Lacanian thought; the animal is already there)—in his discursively elliptical way, he used animals as a means to accentuate, clarify, or illustrate his human-centric psychoanalytic typology, leaving us with a cacophony of digressive fragments or, at times, fleeting full-fledged disquisitions, which can be carefully unified into a Lacanian theory of animality: We can uncover a latent theoretical undercurrent distributed obliquely, but consistently, across his texts. In conjunction with modern scientific research on animals and a philosophical understanding of animality, Lacanian ideas can be deployed to develop a zoological reading of Lacanian theory, and in this book, I intend to enact that unification; *Zoological Lacan* announces, to both the study of animals (in all its variants—from the humanities and the sciences) and psychoanalysis, that a new theory has emerged on the scene, one that warrants substantive and sustained engagement. Psychoanalysis has yet to develop a cogent place for animals, instead opting to cast them as outside the psychoanalytic purview, and other theorists within animal studies, such as Cary Wolfe,[12] have insisted that psychoanalysis structurally forecloses authentic theoretical encounter with the animal mind.

Though Lacan never intended to formulate a theory of animality, his views on animality and humanity expressed throughout his work certainly do not preclude the possibility of his theories being reconfigured in a new capacity oriented to the animal. Even when Lacan is strictly speaking of humans, there is no reason those insights and concepts cannot be repurposed for non-human subjectivity, as long as one accounts for those inherent differences. Lacan himself denied the existence of a "discontinuity" between animals and humans, writing in *Écrits*: "[there is a] misunderstanding of attributing to me the doctrine of a discontinuity between animal psychology and human psychology, which is truly foreign to my way of thinking."[13] Here, it is unmistakable: While Lacan certainly (as we will see in the ensuing chapters) views animals and humans as distinct, there is no reason to totally divorce the study of animals from the study of humans—despite Lacan discussing, almost exclusively, human subjectivity and the unconscious, there is no totalizing discontinuity which forever relegates animals outside the purview of his thought (in the same manner that, although Freud never referenced structuralism, there was an undeniable concurrence between his theories and structuralist ideas that Lacan perceptively detected and could only be retroactively understood).

In this book is a three-pronged procedure I follow to generate an authentic Zoological Lacanian theory, one that holds simultaneous fidelity to both Lacan's ideas and the phenomenology of animality: First, I seek to collate and explicate Lacan's digressive remarks, to enact an interpretive gesture seeking to understand what he means when he refers to animals, and contextualizing this in his overall schema. Second is the partially evaluative element: I compare Lacan's conception of animals to current research on animality. For instance, in Chapter 2, I examine his claim that animals can't recognize themselves in a mirror, and I reference contemporary research that finds that monkeys (and other animals) do have bodily-self-awareness and recognize themselves in the mirror. Through this procedure, I update Lacan's comments on animals (which were made over a half-century ago) according to a modern understanding of animality. Lastly, I generate new insights according to his thoughts on animals and his general psychoanalytic theories that he did not apply to animals—a synthesis of the first two operations. I'm doing this because, with the exception of some articles, no one has applied Lacanian psychoanalysis to animality in book-length form (aside from a single edited collection titled *Lacan and the Nonhuman*)—and I do not think that pure positivism, such as neurology or ethology or biology, exhausts animal subjectivity; I believe animals have an interiority that can come to be known through psychoanalytic insights.

Through enacting this three-pronged approach, I hope to avoid the fate that Lacan polemically consigns to a paper offering a mis-reading of his theories: "[the paper] merits an honorable mention for the art, intentional or otherwise, of taking the consequences of a misunderstanding to their most rigorous conclusions."[14] On two distinct fronts, I plan on evading this "honorable mention" of taking a "misunderstanding to their most rigorous conclusions," both by situating Lacan's comments within his wider theoretical schema and by undoing Lacan's own "misunderstanding" of animality. I cannot promise perfect fidelity to Lacan—there will be departures, especially towards the end through Deleuze and Guattari's conception of the unconscious, but none of these departures will be based on "misunderstanding" his work: They will be intentional deviations necessary to include the animal.

I am hyper-aware of my limitations as a scholar: I am not an ethological researcher; I have never conducted any field research involving animals; nor am I a psychoanalytic clinician. My approach to psychoanalytic theory is closer to philosophy than materialist science (as, I would argue, psychoanalysis—even in its clinical dimension—always has been), and developing a psychoanalytic-philosophical theory of animality necessitates confronting the animal as understood by the discourses of science, which I do not contribute to, but must nonetheless appeal to in order to derive insights reflective of animality. In a different register, the brilliant existentialist theologian Paul Tillich endorses the view that philosophy must rely on empiricism for particular insights into reality: "Just as all sciences have their origin in philosophy, so they contribute in turn to philosophy by giving to the philosopher new and exactly defined material far beyond anything he could get from a prescientific approach to reality."[15] Though I am issuing theoretical assertions in the register of psychoanalytic theory, I must, like the philosopher (or the theologian, as Tillich indicates), extract from science the "new and exactly defined material" that I could not otherwise produce. Lacanian Zoological theory requires contemporary ethological research to ground its claims.

It is crucial to observe, though, that scientific research cannot verify the psychoanalytic claims themselves: They can reject certain claims as 'in contention' with scientific research, but they do not supply the veridicality—or even the true basis—for the claim itself. The claims here are psychoanalytic, which are irreducible to pure scientific empiricism. Conducting physiological tests cannot confirm or deny, for instance, the analytic assertion that dreams are wish-fulfillments. Psychoanalytic case studies could certainly expand, negate, or confirm psychoanalytic claims, but these assertions cannot be confirmed by a brain scan or whatever other neurological tabulation—though, potentially, they could be denied through these processes. Thomas Nagel demonstrates this in his seminal essay on subjectivity, "What Is It Like to Be a Bat?": He writes that when "understanding a phenomenon like lightning, it is legitimate to go as far away as one can from a strictly human viewpoint"[16] because lightning is an event which is "observable from the [human] point of view but external to it."[17] Nagel remains "noncommittal" regarding the "completely objective intrinsic nature of the thing [such as lightning]";[18] despite its intrinsic or non-intrinsic status, the 'objective' phenomenon of lightning can be known without appeal to an individuated viewpoint from which to perceive lightning—lightning can be known through empirical operations that seek to *know* without reference to a specific subjective experience. However, he says that the omission of subjective particularism, a "psychophysical reduction," cannot be applied to understanding subjectivity because "less attachment to a specific viewpoint . . . does not take us nearer to the real nature of the [subjective] phenomenon: it takes us farther away from it."[19]

Subjectivity, such as Nagel's example of the bat's entirely alien interiority, can only be approached with total consideration of the viewpoint in which it subsists. As Nagel writes,

> if the facts of experience—facts about what it is like for the experiencing organisms—are accessible only from one point of view, then it is a mystery how the true character of experiences could be revealed in the physical operation of that organism.[20]

A brain scan, which offers an 'objective' view of the brain's physicality, abstracted from a given experience either *of* or *in* that brain ('of' meaning *observed from without* and 'in' meaning *observed from within*), cannot help us gain much insight into the interior texture of animal subjectivity—but psychoanalysis, with its emphasis on the structure of subjectivity, surely can.

How can animal subjectivity come to be known, if not through objective means? What can psychoanalysis, especially in its Lacanian iteration, contribute to our understanding of animal interiority? Again, we confront the problem of Nagel's essay: The impossibility of embodying another's viewpoint, exacerbated by the experiential gulf animal subjectivity presents. He says, even if we somehow gradually transformed into a bat to understand the bat's phenomenological experiences, "nothing in my present constitution enables me to imagine what the experiences of such a future stage of myself thus metamorphosed would be like."[21] The phenomenological severance between the bat and I (or the cat and I; or the elephant and I; or the insect and I) is total and irrevocable. The problem is, in essence, this: How do we gain intrapsychic knowledge of the animal other through intersubjective means? Near the close of his essay, while attempting to tentatively gesture towards a resolution of this problem, he writes: "structural features of perception might be more accessible to objective description, even though something would be left out."[22] Beyond pure 'imaginative' techniques which attempt to situate us in the place of the animal (such as novel-fiction or poetry or cinema), this is the best method available, even 50 years later, to apprehend animal interiority. What else does psychoanalysis supply, if not this exact mode of explicating the "structural features of perception"? Of taking insights from disparate fields—whether scientific or humanistic—and gleaning a description of subjective processes according to certain principles established by individual cases.

Lacanian psychoanalysis is particularly positioned to do this: Through the triadic topographical structure of the symbolic, imaginary, and the Real, one can situate animals (using research on those "structural features of perceptions") in a psychoanalytic framework. Though it is impossible to occupy their literal 'viewpoint,' animal subjectivity can be known via the psychoanalytic project, which interprets the system of inner-experience (the ostensibly redundant 'inner' is employed here because it is not the experience *of*, but the phenomenological *in* the singular, irreplicable experience). By examining the animal's relation to the symbolic universe (the realm of human language), the imaginary (which I argue, following Lacan, is the structural center of animal subjectivity), and the Real (the encounter with the unmediated space of experience), a properly psychoanalytic theory of animal subjectivity emerges. The first half of the book does exactly this.

The second half of this book synthesizes insights from these three registers—bringing together the Lacanian triad to understand, broadly, two areas of animal interiority: the animal unconscious and human-animal love. In what I anticipate will be the most provocative claim in the book, I assert that animals have an unconscious. However, I situate the animal unconscious as one that operates totally differently from the human unconscious (due to, among other things, human language, with the animal unconscious instead operating according to the imaginary)—and the final definition I offer of this unconscious is, roughly: *activity that must emanate from within* (the animal's subjectivity) *yet posit its activity exogenously, since it issues from the Other*. While I will not entirely explicate it here, I will note that this is clearly distinguished from instinctual activity (since instinctive impulses are *not* issued from the Other). I address the subject of animal love from multiple vantages throughout the book but, in Chapter 5, I arrive at a formulation for the possibility of human-animal love by issuing two aphorisms informed by Lacan's conception of (human-to-human) love: *Loving an animal is giving what we cannot give to one who cannot receive it*, and *we love animals for what they do not have*. As I say in Chapter 5:

> We love animals because we share our lack with them (which they offer back, albeit in a different register), and this love, issued from the unconscious, suffuses their entire being (regardless of the total-whole of their, potentially vulgar or annoying, particularities).

The first three chapters (Part 1), which establish the contours of animal subjectivity according to a Lacanian schema, set the stage for the second half (Part 2), which uses that schema to answer some of the most important subjects of any subjectivity—eros (or a branch of eros: love) and the unconscious. These two subjects are the avowed arenas of psychoanalytic thought, and bringing animals into the psychoanalytic domain necessitates apprehending, however tentatively, their relation to love and the unconscious. It must be said—this is the general texture of animal subjectivity understood broadly: I do not offer access to an individuated, singular animal mind (no psychoanalyst could ever answer the question, *what is this person thinking*, while gazing at a blank face—which is what I anticipate many desire a psychoanalytic book on animality to proffer—nor could they possibly capture all iterations of subjectivity in a single theory; this book does not *psychoanalyze* animals but instead is a psychoanalytic theory of animality); what Zoological Lacanianism offers is a structural mode of understanding individuated animal subjectivities, a theory that works, vertically, from the individual animal (or the species) to the structural features which inform the individual.

In their book, *Wild Justice*, Marc Bekoff and Jessica Pierce cogently warn against the collectivizing effacement of the individuated animal, writing: "One society of animal X may not behave exactly like another society of animal X, and within each society of animal X there are unique individuals each with their own personality and life experiences."[23] The assertion of animal difference must be a guiding principle for approaching animality. As the reader will observe, I write of 'the animal' and 'animality,' nearly universally collapsing all animals into a single classification (which Derrida, the father of 'difference,' would surely have been critical of). Why would I permit myself this gesture of flattening all animals into a single categorization, especially when I am putatively cognizant of the warnings of the theorist and biologist? While I do ensure to classify differences, degrees, and specificities among and between animals, psychoanalysis only functions in generalizations: I cannot say, *here are the particular contours of this cat's interiority* without, in some way, implicating all of animality.

For instance, when Freud wrote a 'case history' focusing on a single patient, such as Dora's, he was not only articulating the contours of their particularized (symptomatic) unconscious emissions and subjectivity but was explicating theoretical premises that underlie all human unconsciousness (and, in the case of Dora, with specific insights towards the nosological category of the hysteric and neuroses). When Freud discusses Dora's first dream (her father waking her and telling her the house is on fire), it is apparent his concern is not only to transmit her case, but also to defend his theory of dream interpretation (the systematic, universalized approach to apprehending the content of dreams). After recounting her dream for the reader, Freud writes, "At this point I shall interrupt my report of the analysis in order to compare this small piece of dream interpretation with the general statements I have made upon the mechanism of the formation of dreams."[24] He then goes on to reconcile her dream with his account of oneiric wish-fulfillment—explaining that the dream was an expression of her ambivalence towards Herr K. (an adult who was effectively preying on her). Freud subsequently declares "the analysis of this dream of Dora's proves afresh that the facts [from the *Interpretation of Dreams*] are as I have supposed."[25] Case histories, for Freud, were not only about the patient, but they also functioned to corroborate or update his always-contested universalized assertions—as he writes, interpreting Dora's dream was "indispensable both for the anamnesis of the case and for the theory of dreams."[26] Psychoanalysis has always oscillated between the individual and the universal, a non-exclusive interchange—but, for the non-clinical theorist (such as myself), this oscillation is in service of the theory exceeding the individual (but, to ensure its veridicality, must remain attached to the study of individual animals).

Animality does, of course, present new difficulties not yet contended with by psychoanalysis. Namely, the difficulty of establishing psychoanalytic theories applicable *across species*—it will strike many as dubious to bring together the ant and the elephant under the banner of a common psychoanalytic theory. In a sense, this instinct is correct: there is no reason to believe an ant and an elephant, with entirely dissimilar perceptual systems, have the same inner-experience of the world (or even to assume two elephants have the same experience). We can broadly assert both the ant and the elephant do not have access to the symbolic (they do not deploy signifiers which hold an arbitrary relation to that which they signify, sliding across disparate signifieds) and, consequently, we can assert that their subjectivity must be mediated by the imaginary (though the qualities of their respective imaginaries, refracted through perception, are surely distinct). Then, we can assert that there are fleeting moments which puncture the mediating surface of the imaginary, bringing a requisite traumatic encounter or jouissance (enjoyment-beyond-pleasure) which exceeds comprehension (comprehension here referring to the mediating field refracting reality)—and, in the case of trauma, this is clearly something that occurs across discrete species (as I demonstrate in Chapter 3), from rats to primates and elephants. At this juncture-site, where disparate species meet in a common experiential domain, it seems appropriate to refer to *animality*—while keeping in mind that this primarily refers to social mammals. Tediously listing out each applicable species would be a scientific fantasy; imaginary subjectivity is clearly something applicable across a range of animality, which I delineate throughout this book. (It would undoubtedly supply indispensable insights if one applied Zoological Lacanianism to a single species, examining the attributes of a given *kind* of animal—or perhaps there would be even more utility in applying this to a case study of an individual animal, generating a psychoanalytic profile of their interiority; a case history of a cat named 'Dora,' rather than a young adult girl. How one would conduct this is unclear to me and would surely be handled better by a clinical psychoanalyst.)

The true contribution of Zoological Lacanianism is opening up a topological approach to animal subjectivity, one refusing to cast aside animals as unknowable, and in the same gesture, declining to collapse animality into humanity—it is a theoretical approach that takes human-animal difference seriously in order to, very carefully, extricate the animal from beneath the mammoth of writings and research on the human. Freud, in his book *Jokes and Their Relation to the Unconscious*, declares that

> In the realization that we are standing upon ground which has never been trodden [in studying the unconscious], we are thus content, from our point of observation, to take one single, short and uncertain step forward into the unexplored region.[27]

When studying the "unexplored region" of animal subjectivity, we must similarly be "content" with our "uncertain step forward." We have just begun to incorporate the fact, made evident over the last few decades, that animals have subjectivity, but have frequently denied ourselves any knowledge of the content of this subjectivity for fear of committing the dreaded *anthropomorphism*, leading the stream of psychoanalytic knowledge to eschew the site of the animal, like an obstructive rock in a flowing river. *Zoological Lacan* is a movement in that direction—towards the site of the animal—and through this, we learn that accepting the fact of animal subjectivity should not convince us animals are more like us but rather that they are incomprehensibly different. Just as we all are, when encountered by an-other.

Notes

1 Jacques Lacan, *Écrits*, trans. Bruce Fink (New York: W. W. Norton & Company, 2006), 203.
2 Jacques Lacan, *The Ethics of Psychoanalysis: The Seminar of Jacques Lacan, Book VII*, ed. Jacques-Alain Miller, trans. Dennis Porter (New York: W. W. Norton & Company, 1992), 37.
3 Jacques Lacan, *The Formations of the Unconscious: The Seminar of Jacques Lacan, Book V*, ed. Jacques-Alain Miller, trans. Russell Grigg (Cambridge: Polity Press, 2017), 74.
4 Jonathan Dickstein and Gautam Thakur, eds., *Lacan and the Nonhuman* (New York: Palgrave Macmillan, 2017), 3–4.
5 Andrew Spicer, "L'extermination de tout Symbolisme des Cieux: Reading the Lacanian Letter as Inhuman 'Apparatus' and Its Implications for Ecological Thinking," in *Lacan and the Nonhuman*, ed. Jonathan Dickstein and Gautam Thakur (New York: Palgrave Macmillan, 2017), 104.
6 Lacan, *Formations of the Unconscious*, 64.
7 Katie Gentile, "Animals as the Symptom of Psychoanalysis or, the Potential for Interspecies Co-Emergence in Psychoanalysis," *Studies in Gender and Sexuality* 19, no. 1 (2018): 8.
8 Gentile, "Animals as the Symptom of Psychoanalysis or, the Potential for Interspecies Co-Emergence in Psychoanalysis," 8.
9 Gentile, "Animals as the Symptom of Psychoanalysis or, the Potential for Interspecies Co-Emergence in Psychoanalysis," 8.
10 Jacques Lacan, *The Four Fundamental Concepts of Psycho-Analysis: The Seminar of Jacques Lacan, Book XI*, ed. Jacques-Alain Miller, trans. Alan Sheridan (New York: W. W. Norton & Company, 1981), 230.
11 Charles Shepherdson, "Lacan and Philosophy," in *The Cambridge Companion to Lacan*, ed. Jean-Michel Rabaté (Cambridge: Cambridge University Press, 2003), 125.
12 See Cary Wolfe, *Animal Rites: American Culture, the Discourse of Species, and Posthumanist Theory* (Chicago: University of Chicago Press, 2003).
13 Lacan, *Écrits*, 404.
14 Lacan, *Écrits*, 205.
15 Paul Tillich, *Systematic Theology*, Vol. 1 (Chicago: University of Chicago Press, 1951), 12.
16 Thomas Nagel, *What Is It Like to Be a Bat?* (Oxford: Oxford University Press, 2024), 18.
17 Nagel, *What Is It Like to Be a Bat?*, 17.
18 Nagel, *What Is It Like to Be a Bat?*, 17.
19 Nagel, *What Is It Like to Be a Bat?*, 20.

20 Nagel, *What Is It Like to Be a Bat?*, 16.
21 Nagel, *What Is It Like to Be a Bat?*, 10.
22 Nagel, *What Is It Like to Be a Bat?*, 28.
23 Marc Bekoff and Jessica Pierce, *Wild Justice: The Moral Lives of Animals* (Chicago: University of Chicago Press, 2009), 20.
24 Sigmund Freud, *Dora: Fragment of an Analysis of a Case of Hysteria*, trans. James Strachey (Touchstone, 1997), 59.
25 Freud, "Dora," 78.
26 Freud, "Dora," 63.
27 Sigmund Freud, *Jokes and Their Relation to the Unconscious*, trans. James Strachey (New York: W. W. Norton & Company, 1989), 220.

Part 1

Animal Subjects in the Lacanian Triad (The Symbolic, the Imaginary, and the Real)

Chapter 1

Lacan's Rats

The Limits of Language in Animal Subjectivity

Although Jacques Lacan's work—particularly his earlier seminars—contains remarks on ethology, and he has other semi-consistent but fleeting references to animality, such as his contention that 'shit' is the line that demarcates animality from human civilization, the famous reflection on pigeons and the mirror stage, or his passing observations on the relation of 'the animal' to the signifier, there is not a sustained, explicit engagement with the 'animal question.' Oftentimes, animals were used to illuminate his true subject—the human unconscious—by distinguishing animal subjectivity and human subjectivity. He certainly never developed a systematic psychoanalytic approach to animals. In a certain sense, he foreclosed the possibility of a robust confrontation with animal subjects. In his seminar VII, *The Ethics of Psychoanalysis*, he resolutely states that there is a fundamental, constitutive unknowability to animals that cannot be "resolved in psychological terms":

> When we seek to explore the frontier between the animal and the human world, it is apparent to what extent the symbolic process as such doesn't function in the animal world . . . . That man is caught up in symbolic processes of a kind to which no animal has access cannot be resolved in psychological terms, since it implies that we first have a complete and precise knowledge of what this symbolic process means.[1]

Here, Lacan indicates an awareness of the epistemic problem which animals present for psychoanalysis and—rather than merely dismissing the animal question as unworthy of further investigation—he determines that there is a central intractability to the question that cannot be dissolved through psychoanalytic inquiry. For Lacan, knowledge of the human-animal frontier, and what it means to be an animal without access (or limited access) to the symbolic, is marked by impossibility due to the necessarily incomplete (human) knowledge of the "symbolic process" itself. Yet, as we will see, this does not relegate animals to some entirely sealed-off inaccessible domain of non-knowledge—there is still a possibility for a schematic Lacanian approach to animality.

The question concerning Lacan and animals is not (or, rather, should not be): *How might we render animal subjectivity transparent through psychoanalysis and*

DOI: 10.4324/9781003635383-3

gain unmediated access to their internality? As Lacanian psychoanalysis insists, even human subjectivity is never transparent, and is instead revealed through small escapes facilitated by the signifier which emerges by interventions from "what lies beyond the subject"[2]—the unconscious. Simply, the unconscious uses language through substitution (metonymy and metaphor) to generate a cyphered message—and, notably, these messages are not transparent to the subject. We see this in the most elementary case of parapraxis or negation: The subject does not know what they say; they think the escaped signifier is merely a meaningless mistake that signifies nothing more than a motor-functional failure. Therefore, if humans, as those who wield the signifier (which, as a communicative apparatus, should ostensibly enable the clear transmission of concepts and feeling) do not have direct unmediated access to others or even to ourselves, then we cannot reasonably expect animal subjectivity (whatever that may be, in a psychoanalytic sense) to transparently display itself. Accordingly, the proper question regarding animality is, instead: *What can be said about the limit that animals present to the symbolic? What can be known about the abyss of animal subjectivity?* We should not expect, nor should we ever expect with Lacan, a direct response—but rather an oblique response, to a domain (animality) which is itself oblique and indirect, language-less (or to be precise, signifier-less), and must be approached hermeneutically.

The concluding lecture of Seminar XX, titled "The Rat in the Maze," presents one of Lacan's most immediate confrontations with animality—specifically animality's relation to love, knowledge, and, as I will argue, the symbolic. In the seminar, Lacan explores epistemological questions—along with the body, jouissance, and love—through the prism of a study of rats within a maze. I assert that a thorough reading of this small chapter, conjoined with Lacan's other statements on animals, can provide a starting silhouette, a tracing, of the Lacanian perspective on the animal-human 'frontier' in terms of language—an outlook that is not merely significant for Lacanians or the study of psychoanalysis, but also has substantive implications for general animal studies.

Lacan and Behaviorism: The Relation of Human (Signifier) to Animal (Sign)

To approach Lacan's conception of animality, we must first analyze Lacan's view of behaviorism: it is immediately pertinent to a study of his conception of animality because the behavioral approach (popular during Lacan's time) took animals as its subject in order to derive insights that are putatively applicable to humans or generalizable. Lacan repeatedly explicates the failure of psychological behaviorism in his work, undermining its underlying theoretical framework of positivist science and its implicit dismissal of the unconscious and its language-structure. For Lacan (and many other prominent thinkers, such as Noam Chomsky in his review of B.F. Skinner's book),[3] behaviorism represents a naive positivist-materialist methodology that refuses to situate language—and even consciousness—within its proper place in relation to human thought and behavior. As Freud wrote of behaviorism's rejection of analyzing consciousness: "the American doctrine of behaviourism, thinks it possible to construct a psychology which disregards this fundamental fact [of consciousness]!"[4] It is a methodology, which Lacan frequently addressed through sharp criticisms, that explores the human-animal boundary by extrapolating from animal behavior to conclusions about humans. By understanding Lacan's criticisms of behaviorism, which is a key dimension of "The Rat in the Maze," we can begin to approach the general Lacanian view of the human-animal boundary in the symbolic domain.

In a much earlier seminar, Seminar V, Lacan comments on the quintessential behaviorist: Ivan Pavlov. According to Lacan, the basic Pavlovian experiments subjected animals to a system predicated on language, yet the animals themselves did not have access to the language-system that they were embedded in. All the methods Pavlov and other behaviorists rely on, like the famous "little bells," to induce physiological responses like salivation, are "all the same signifiers."[5] In other words, as Hub Zwart observes, the Pavlovian laboratory is, for Lacan, a "symbolic environment"[6] deploying signifiers to generate a physical response. Yet, notably, Lacan declares that "when all is said and done, [Pavlov's conditioned reflex] does not amount to teaching these animals who are so well trained a certain type of language."[7] Behaviorism is thus a practice that subjects animals to a domain (the symbolic) which they cannot fully penetrate, then extracts insights about animals from these symbolic experiments (that are later anemically applied to humans). For animals, the signifiers (such as the bell that functions as a signifier for food) are rendered mere 'signals'—they are nothing but signs.

This sign/signifier distinction is a system that, for Lacan, defines the respective positions of animals and humans in relation to language and largely defines the status of their subjectivity. He explains this postulation in "The Rat in the Maze":

> The only thing the rat-unit learns in this case is to give a sign, a sign of its presence as unit. The flap is recognized only by a sign and pressing its paw on this sign is a sign. It is always by making a sign that the unit accedes to that on the basis of which one concludes that there is learning. But this relation to signs is external. Nothing confirms that the rat grasps the mechanism to which pressing the button leads.[8]

Here, Lacan denies the basic discovery of behaviorism: These experiments do not indicate animal learning (in terms of a proper engagement in the symbolic: an apprehension of signifiers) since the animal does not deploy "the flap" as a signifier but instead as a sign. The relation remains external—the "rat," in this case, remains tethered to the outward appearance of the function of the sign—apprehension of the flap's "mechanism" eludes the rat. In other words, nothing about the rat pressing the flap with its paw indicates anything at all regarding the interiority of the rat, aside from its recognition that the flap will provide food. One could only prove that the rat 'learned' if those observing the animal determined, from the rat's external behavior, that there had been an intellectual augmentation of some kind—that the rat grasped the 'meaning' of the flap beyond it being the ineffable material somehow causing the pellet's manifestation. Of course, there is some internal functioning that corresponds to the external mechanism (of determining that the flap will generate food)—but this is far from comprehending the nature of the flap *as a signifier.* Lacan does not object to the fact that the little rat figures out the flap will produce food, instead positing that the rat does not learn "the mechanism to which pressing the bottom leads." An understanding of the mechanism is the arena of the symbolic—of knowing the flap as a signifier rather than a sign.

Why is this little flap, which is for humans a signifier, instead a sign for the rat? Is the sign/signifier severance not just an anthropocentric non-distinction that reifies pre-conceptions of animality? If one looks closely, the signifier turns out to be a distinct concept from the sign in crucial ways: the signifier, unlike the sign, holds an arbitrary relation to the signifier. The arbitrary relation between signifier and signified—an insight popularized by Saussurean linguistics that informed structuralist, and subsequently Lacanian, thought—is the basic defining matrix of human language. Lacan states, in the same vein as Saussure, that there is a "certain impenetrability" that maintains the "distance between the signifier and the signified."[9] A signifier's distance, generated by an "impenetrability," suggests a relationship that cannot be collapsed: there cannot be, as Lacan says of the sign, an immediate, non-arbitrary relation between the signifier and the signified.

In *Écrits*, Lacan directly confronts the issue of animal language—commenting on Karl von Frisch's ethological research into bee 'language.' Here, again, he clearly designates animal "language" as a sign:

> It is now generally recognized that, when a bee returns to its hive after gathering nectar, it transmits an indication of the existence of nectar near or far away from the hive to its companions by two sorts of dances. The second is the most remarkable, for the plane in which the bee traces out a figure-eight—a shape that gave it the name "wagging dance"—and the frequency of the figures executed within a given time, designate, on the one hand, the exact direction to be followed, determined in relation to the sun's inclination (by which bees are able to orient themselves in all kinds of weather, thanks to their sensitivity to polarized light), and, on the other hand, the distance at which the nectar is to be found up to several miles away. The other bees respond to this message by immediately setting off for the place thus designated . . . . But is it a language, for all that? We can say that it is distinguished from language precisely by the fixed correlation between its signs and the reality they signify. For, in a language, signs take on their value from their relations to each other.[10]

A similar formula is re-produced here, albeit Lacan is relying on a distinct vocabulary from his later seminar on "Rats in the Maze": animal "language" (which he later says is predicated on signs) is fixed in its "correlation" to the inertia of reality; while human language (which he postulates as predicated on the signifier) is non-contingent on a reality-correlation. As Lacan insists, the constitutive mark of the signifier is its very severance from objective reality and the signified. Rather than being language, this communicative gesture bees emit—the "wagging dance"—is "a code or signaling system."[11] Language (the signifier), conversely, adheres to no such inflexibly binding code. The dance, although containing a message, is "frozen in its function as a relay of action" and never "becomes a symbol of communication itself."[12] The dance is a pure signified—the bee could not conceive of producing this dance in the absence of a corresponding action, and neither could there be any ambiguity in the dance aside from a potential malfunction, a mis-dance. Later, in the "Seminar on the 'Purloined Letter'" Lacan unequivocally relegates the bee act as a "supposed language" that merely is the "signaling of the location of object."[13]

Yet, there remains a lingering objection: How can the same object (the little flap) be considered both a 'sign' and a 'signifier'? The object itself, of course, has nothing to do with its status as either sign or signifier—only through its relation to a 'subject' does the flap become more than an inert thing. For the human, the flap is a signifier because it is bound up in signifieds that exceed its function as a flap—the flap is not merely something which flaps, or 'generates' pellets (as it is for the rat); it is, instead, known in its interrelation to other signifiers within the symbolic. The flap is, for the human behaviorist researcher, a word in all its materiality, in all its non-transparent, flexible relationality—meaning the signifier 'flap' consists of four letters and is distinguished from 'flag' due to the placement of the final letter; the individual signifier occupies a position in relation to other signifiers that make up the lexicon available to the subject. For the human researcher, the flap does not enter into a direct equation such as *flap = sustenance*, but rather a differential relation to other phonetically similar signifiers ('flag,' 'flop'); other representationally similar signifiers ('button,' 'lever'); and other unconsciously tethered signifiers, like in the instance of someone that encountered a flap during a particular traumatic event, who may substitute the term for something seemingly unrelated that constitutes an unconscious relationship, in order to not endure a confrontation with a traumatic event. A signifier is only known in the negative—as is the thing it signifies (the signified). In short, the signifier means much more for the researcher than *that which brings nourishment*—which is the exact meaning (if it can be called 'meaning') it holds for the rat. For the experiment itself, the flap is a signifier that represents much more than merely a button to be pressed: it is bound up in its meaning within the experiment itself, as that which indicates, for the researchers, success or failure.

Lacan defines the "essential property of the signifier" as the fact that "something can intervene that makes of its signifiers disappear and puts another signifier in its place"[14] within the signifying chain. It is the "essential polyvalence and creative function," along with "the touch of the arbitrary"[15] that the signifier brings, which generates human meaning. Definitionally, signifiers can be substituted for one another. Substitution—and more specifically metaphor, an indispensable concept for Lacan—is the basic function of the signifier and allows the cryptic emergence of the unconscious, engendered by the arbitrary signifier/signified relation. Metaphor, in Lacan's thought, is the act of an unconscious signifier taking the place of a conscious one in speech (or writing). He unambiguously declares that the "multiplication of significations that characterize the enriching of the human world" originates in the "substitution of a signifier for another signifier."[16] The entire psychoanalytic project of 'free association' is contingent on the unconscious metaphoric substitution of signifiers. If there was a direct correspondence between signifier and signified (as he argues there is for animals), then substitution would be a null concept; there would be no substitution, or 'sliding' among signifiers because each signifier would miraculously correspond to its given signified. This is precisely why Lacan explicates that "the supposed language of certain animals" is a "sign language which neither allows for metaphor nor engenders metonymy."[17]

In a sense, we can already detect a major (symbolic) difference between animals and humans: animals cannot be approached, psychoanalytically, in the same fashion as humans, due to this irreconcilable sign/signifier distinction—the sign has an immediate relation to that which it signals, and the signifier, as a linguistic unit—a word—does not. In psychoanalysis, consciousness, and more importantly, unconsciousness, emerges through speech (and the signifier in general); without this dimension—the dimension of the symbolic, which Lacan only confers to humans—it is literally impossible to access the interiority of any given animal, even more impossible than it is to reach the interiority of another human, or even ourselves. This is exactly what Lacan means, in the quote at the start of this chapter, when he asserts that "man is caught up in symbolic processes of a kind to which no animal has access"[18] and that, in order to "resolve" this meaning, we would need a complete knowledge of that symbolic process, which he claims we do not have. Precisely because we do not have unmediated access to each other, despite having language (being 'in' the symbolic), along with the fact that we must *remain* within the symbolic, never going 'outside' of it, precludes our knowledge of animals—the animal question is thus a compounded variant of the human question.

The perceptive reader may assert that Lacan's work is caught in a certain reductiveness at this juncture—a thoughtless replication of the same philosophically-sanctioned binary position of animality and humanity which has plagued the conception of both the animal and the human. How, if he is not replicating—by default—those philosophical presuppositions, does the sign/signifier distinction avoid a binary division forever severing animality and humanity? Does this site of difference (the inflexible animal sign and the constitutively supple human signifier) not comport itself with the orthodox view of animals as languageless and humans as exceptional (and thus superior) in their deployment of language? It is certainly true—since it is a point that he insists on again and again—that in Lacanian thought the animal is languageless (in the sense defined so far, of human language constituted by the symbolic and the signifier). But Lacan does not deny that the bees' act is a communicative gesture—the dance does, unequivocally, operate on the plane of communication. The bees' dance makes its way into Lacan's texts precisely because it is an act of animal communication which he identifies as such. Animal studies scholar Sean Meighoo, in his article "Human Language, Animal Code, and the Question of Being," concludes that this is the wrong view of Lacan's position on animal language:

> [In] Lacan's work, while both the human and the animal possess the capacity for communication, the human and at least one kind of nonhuman animal—the bee—are capable of communication by code or a system of signals whereas the human alone is further capable of communication by language or a system of symbols. Human language and animal code, then, do not comprise mutually exclusive domains or capacities.[19]

Meighoo notes in the following paragraph that, for thinkers like Lacan (which he calls "structuralist"), "the human and the animal are distinguished not along the lines of a simple binary opposition but rather in the more flexible terms of an 'exception'."[20] In Lacan's work, there is not a simplified binary, despite the fact that it maintains a crucial—and irrevocable—*difference*.

There is no division between non-communicative animals and communicative humans—it is, rather, a spectrum of communicativity with humans relying on language-communication and animals relying on code-communication. Animal code and human language are thus points of difference, both residing in an operative continuum of *communication*, without functioning as "mutually exclusive domains." Human language is exceptional in the same way bee code is exceptional, relying on distinct communicative materials and procedures. Both modalities of communication have their own implications for the 'subjects' that deploy them. For Lacan, the use of the signifiers is, according to Meighoo, "a singular emergence of vital upsurge from the immanent field of being."[21] The human capacity for the signifier and the symbolic is 'singular' but not conceived of as a 'simple binary opposition.'

Lacan's insight that the same object (in the case mentioned previously, a flap) is a sign for the animal (the rat) but a signifier for a human (the a researcher) brings us back to the deficiencies he identifies with behaviorism: not only is behaviorism fundamentally incapable of supplying substantive knowledge regarding humans, but he also much more radically contests its utility in even elucidating much about animal interiority. This modality of knowledge can be compared to the function of a lie detector—the lie detector is a device that apprises us of certain physiological processes and disjunctors in the subject (a rising in blood pressure and stress levels), yet truly offers no insight into the interiority of the subject's consciousness: A lie detector, like behaviorism, remains tethered to the external representations (signifiers transmitted to the researchers)—meaning internal phenomena (where the lie is 'contained') maintain their alterity and unknowability despite the lie detectors unfulfilled promise of transparent access to the internal through external significations. Behaviorism apprises us of the researcher's subjectivity more than animals or other humans who act as subjects to their experiments. Peter Buse writes in his article "The Dog and the Parakeet: Lacan Among the Animals," that "In [Lacan's] *Encore*, the maze the experimenter lays out for the rat—its tests, its punishments, its rewards—does not yield up data about the rat's reaction and response, but about the knowledge and desire of the experiment."[22] Behaviorism and the myth of the lie detector operate according to this same collapsing of the internal and external—claiming that interiority can be reached via external manifestations.

The Status of Animal(s) Knowledge and the Capacity to Lie Via Truth

If behaviorism presents us with a failed methodology for understanding animal subjectivity, then how can we come to know the status of animal knowledge? Further, the concern for animal knowledge is compounded by the cacophony of texts, from various disciplines, that promulgate or even unequivocally prove animals' ability to engage in what we broadly refer to as language. Some of these texts, as we will see, even respond directly to Lacan's perspective of animals' status as signifier-less. These texts, many of them excellent studies, seem to negate the sign/signifier distinction—animals are found to use language in nuanced and complicated ways. Human language, seen from this vantage, is one particular modality of language among many. Lacan's answer to both of these questions is somewhat unexpected and unorthodox: the human capacity to pretend to tell the truth, to lie and have awareness that one is lying and present the lie as if it were true—not just to conceal but to conceal through falsehood in the register of truth, or as Derrida writes, to "*pretend to pretend*"[23]—is one of the most telling attributes of the conditions which designate our language and knowledge as distinctly 'human.'

Typically, the dividing line that separates animality and humanity—humans being viewed as a hyper-distinct species, not because every species is distinguishable from others due to particular attributes and idiosyncrasies, but rather in a deeper, more entrenched sense of humans being radically severed from the realm of animality—is language.[24] It is tempting to assign this same commonplace, and slightly asinine, view to Lacan—especially considering that Freud posited "the function of speech" as an "added complication"[25] that animals did not need to contend with in their conscious experience. Yet, putting aside Freud's statement (we should not necessarily interpret his quote as entirely capitulating to the presupposition that animals are languageless), it is clear Lacan did not totally preclude animals from the domain of language, but instead precludes them, reasonably enough, as we have seen, from comprehension of and proper participation in the symbolic universe contingent on the signifier's function.

Lacan poses that animals can partake in language through the vocalized (or, in certain cases, non-vocalized) transmittal of messages, noting that "You have only to observe a pet to see that a being deprived of language is quite capable of making calls on you, calls to draw your attention to something which, in some sense or other, it lacks."[26] This 'call' that Lacan refers to is certainly a communicative mode—whether it is the bark of the dog to signal they need to go outside to urinate, or an inter-species transmission of aggression, such as two feral cats encountering each other in the street and viscously hissing. According to the apparatus of communicative vocalization (or gestural non-vocalization), we can ascertain, as other fields have, that animals have language. Crucially, though, Lacan claims that animals are "deprived of language"—yet, for a simple resolution of the animal problem, we should take what Lacan calls "language" to mean human language, the language he is concerned with in the psychoanalytic sense, the language that operates within the symbolic field with all the implications that comes with that field, as enumerated in the preceding section.

The assertion that animals are not deprived of language (understood as a means of communicative transmission) but instead are deprived of the signifier seems to bring us no closer than the last section on the sign/signifier distinction in understanding animal knowledge—and this is exactly why we must return to Lacan's contention regarding animals' capacity to lie. In "The Subversion of the Subject and the Dialectic of Desire," Lacan writes the following essential passage:

> [A]n animal does not feign feigning. It does not make tracks whose deceptiveness lies in getting them to be taken as false, when in fact they are true—that is, tracks that indicate the right trail. No more than it effaces its tracks, which would already be tantamount to making itself the subject of the signifier.[27]

Lacan claims an animal cannot, in Derrida's words, "pretend to pretend"; they cannot pretend they are pretending during the presentation of truth, a second order of pretending that necessitates distinguishing between pretend and truth, leveraging the appearance of one over the other. Earlier in the same essay, he describes that animals *do* have the capacity to "feign": "animals show that they are capable of such behavior when they are being hunted down; they manage to throw their pursuers off the scent by briefly going in one direction as a lure and then changing direction."[28] Simply, animals can attempt to deceive; they are able to lie and conceal, but they are incapable of presenting a truth as if it were a lie—pretending that the truth is a lie in order to conceal the lie within the truth qua truth.

To provide an example of the conventional modality of deception, of the first layer of animal feigning: think of the domestic dog who engages in explicitly prohibited behavior—the Law of the household. How does the dog act in this instance? Do they not attempt to conceal the act, for instance by eluding the human once they enter the scene? We could view this, though, as the animal simply avoiding consequences due to instincts—the avoidance of punitive judgment through flight. Yet we also see instances of dogs deliberately 'feigning' as if they did not commit the act: a dog who urinates or defecates in the house, who subsequently avoids the location of the excrement, continuing as if the act against a known injunction had not been committed. Or consider the dog who 'steals' another pet's toy or food and hides it—they have awareness that the 'stolen' object is clearly designated as another's, leading to the necessity of the deceitful concealment. We can infer from these foregoing examples that animals can feign—they are capable, as Lacan says, of taking a trail then deceptively cutting into another 'direction.' This is precisely why Lacan attributes to dogs a "superego": "dogs are exceptions in the sense that, although they do not have an unconscious, they have a superego."[29] Lying—not merely evading danger or simply fleeing but decidedly concealing an act—indicates that we may be contending with (a modality of) superegoic guilt.

We have not only concluded, following Lacan, that animals can feign; we have also precluded animals from feigning to feign, or 'feign feigning.' Referencing again the example of an animal being pursued, Lacan claims an animal cannot make the true 'tracks' appear false, trying to throw the pursuer off the chase by somehow convincing them that they have changed direction when they haven't, such as deliberately covering their paw prints to implicate another direction (thereby erasing the trace of their presence)—they cannot present the truth as if it was false—and, notably, if they could do so, that would render them, according to Lacan, a 'subject of the signifier.' How does this secondary layer of feigning, of lying or pretending, become so consequential and relate to the operation of the signifier and the symbolic order? It is the split, the necessary division, between the subject of enunciation and the subject of the statement that determines the signifier's significance. There is the grammatical, self-reflexive 'I' of the sentence and the subject who speaks/writes that I—the one from whom the sentence issues. This is how a statement such as 'I am lying' emerges as paradoxical: there is the inherent severance between the grammatical 'I' who is stated as 'lying' and the speaking or writing subject who is declaring that they are not lying—that they are disclosing the truth about lying. Yet, Lacan contends, "It is clear that the *I am lying* despite its paradox, is perfectly valid. Indeed, the *I* of the enunciation is not the same as the *I* of the statement."[30] 'I am lying' exhibits the very basis of 'feign feigning': one is either telling the truth via a lie or lying via the truth. Simply, the signifier enables the subject (of the signifier) to generate statements such as these—statements which can lie through the truth by relying on the subject's awareness. A dog or cat could never issue a statement such as 'I am lying'; they cannot conceivably communicate an utterance that contains an inextricable convergence of truth and lie. They cannot convince an-other that the tracks going in the correct direction are falsely-false.

For Lacan, the meaning of the signifier's function is partially that it subsists on this severance—an irreducible gap—between truth and lie, between the materiality of the signifier and content it carries (with the potentiality of a lie surfacing from this fundamental misalignment). This is the gap, of course, that introduces the psychoanalytic method: not only can the subject use the signifier to cover their own 'tracks'—by using the signifier to lie under a guise of truth—the unconscious relies on this same structure to facilitate its own emergence. This is precisely why Lacan, in what may seem a paradoxical statement, writes that "speech is inscribed in truth even when it lies."[31] The truth exists, inexorably, in speech through the procedure of substitution—and its relation to the subject of enunciation. Consider, for instance, parapraxis: the signifier of the unconscious emerges under the guise of an accidental slip of the tongue (an unconscious 'truth' percolates up into speech under the guise of a lie). For a classic Freudian example: One means to say to the analyst, 'My *wife* and I are in deep, passionate love, but I feel I cannot have sex with her.' Instead, the analysand remarks, 'My *mother* and I are in deep, passionate love, but I feel I cannot have sex with her.' The unconscious uses the intrinsic substitution of the signifier to enact the epitome of pretending to pretend: the truth emerges in the form of a slip (a lie) to be veiled (the 'tracks' covered) under the guise of an inadvertent slip-of-the-tongue. Of course, when the analysand said mother, what they *really* meant is mother (albeit the analysand will claim what they 'really meant' was wife, and that the utterance-slip was entirely motor-functional). Truth emerges in the form of a false-mistake.

Consider another classic Freudian instantiation of lying via truth, a joke which has no explicit relation to the unconscious:

> Two Jews met in a railway carriage at a station in Galicia. 'Where are you going?' asked one. 'To Cracow', was the answer. 'What a liar you are!' broke out the other. 'If you say you're going to Cracow, you want me to believe you're going to Lemberg. But I know that in fact you're going to Cracow. So why are you lying to me?'[32]

Evidently, the subject who asks the question, "Where are you going?" already knows the answer (the other is going to Cracow)—and the joke lies in the fact that the questioner accuses the other of 'lying' precisely because he tells the truth. The questioner expects the other to misdirect them by lying (to claim they are going to X so the other believes they're going to Y), and this expectation leads them to consider the truth a lie (to claim they are going to X, thinking the other will believe they are going to Y, when they are actually, in reality, going to X). As Freud explains, "according to the uncontradicted assertion of the first Jew, the second is lying when he tells the truth and is telling the truth by means of a lie."[33] Here, we find the second-order deception of 'feigning to feign': A deception which accounts for the other's expectations regarding truth. *The other will expect me to lie* (to say that I'm going to Y when I'm really going to X); *therefore, I must be truthful to deceive them* (to tell them I'm going to X when I'm actually going to X, since they will believe I'm going to Y). How is this distinct from a conventional lie? A conventional lie would be, *I'm going to X* (*but really, I'm going to Y*). However, because the other knows the questioner expects them to lie, a lie such as this would not work: They must tell the truth in an attempt to doubly misdirect the questioner. The joke is, effectively, that lie and truth become indistinguishable; either way the second Jew will be under suspicion of lying. There is absolutely nothing in animality that implicates them in this second order of deception-via-truth. An animal either feigns or does not feign, lies or tells the truth.

Lacan's distinction between feigning and feigning to feign has certainly not gone uncontested. In his seminal text on animals, *The Animal That Therefore I am*, Derrida replies to Lacan's assertion that animals cannot 'feign feigning':

> The status of the affirmation that refuses the pretense of pretense to the animal is that of a simple dogma. But there is no doubt a dissimulated motivation to this humanist or anthropocentric dogmatism, and that is the probably obscure

> but indisputable feeling that it is indeed difficult, even impossible, to discern between pretense and a pretense of pretense, between an aptitude for pretense and an aptitude for the pretense of pretense. How could one distinguish, for example, in the most elementary sexual mating game, between a feint and a feint of a feint? If it here provides the criterion for such a distinction, one can conclude that every pretense of pretense remains a simple pretense (animal or imaginary, in Lacan's terms) or else, on the contrary, and just as likely, that every pretense, however simple it may be, gets repeated and reposited undecidably, in its possibility, as pretense of pretense (human or symbolic in Lacan's terms).[34]

Derrida contends here that Lacan provides no 'ethological' evidence for his postulation that animals cannot 'feign feigning' or—as he puts it—the claim that they cannot operate under the 'pretense of a pretense.' For Derrida, Lacan's claims are nothing but a reification of a philosophical bias (anthropocentrism) that denies psychoanalytic theory itself, since, as he writes, "a symptomatology (and, of course, a psychoanalysis) can and must conclude with the possibility, for every pretense, of being pretense of pretense."[35] He contests the assumption that one can discern the difference between *pretending* and *pretending to pretend*—and claims that psychoanalytic theory itself does not allow for the preclusion of the secondary layer to any communicative utterance. Derrida asserts psychoanalysis is predicated on the fact that "every erased trace, in consciousness, can leave a trace of its erasure"[36] through the symptom which can always return. For the human, the trace is never erased (due to its return, possibly in the unconscious), and for animals we can never know if the trace was erased since, for Derrida, "the structure of the trace presupposes that to *trace* amounts to *erasing a trace*."[37] A trace, the remainder the subject leaves behind, is an absence indicative of a former presence—the subject is present via an absence.

It is likely apparent here to the scrupulous reader that Derrida is no longer referring to the literal-material 'tracks' that Lacan was relying on as an example—he has now moved onto his (related) famous concept of the 'trace' as the principal feature of signification. Although this may seem unrelated to Lacan's initial claim, it should be recalled that Lacan's primary insight was that the ability to cover tracks, to feign feigning—what Derrida calls a "second-degree reflexive power, a power that is *conscious* of deceiving"[38]—is what renders one a 'subject of the signifier.' Both Lacan and Derrida's analysis of the lying of animals is intimately tied to language-usage and signification. Derrida, though, seems to be indicating that animals either are 'subjects of the signifier' or at least cannot be categorically excluded from such a status (that they *could be* subjects of the signifier)—he refuses, in either case, to determinatively exhaust the interiority of animals. He rejects the proposition not only that animals are incapable of 'feign feigning' but also that we can *know* if animals can feign feigning.

Although Derrida's commentary appears to undermine Lacan's claim of animals being precluded from a distinct modality of language-usage—that we nominally call *human* language, and Lacan calls 'the symbolic' and predicates on the function of the signifier—his challenge merely modifies, or more precisely delineates, the Lacanian perspective. Derrida's contention can be split into two categories: an epistemological critique and a linguistic-psychoanalytic critique. As stated in the preceding paragraph, Derrida is calling into question both what can be known about animals and the ethological reality of animal consciousness and communication. In terms of the epistemological critique—where Derrida issues a challenge of how Lacan *knows* that a given animal cannot pretend to pretend or consciously deceive—it is a perfectly reasonable inquiry: "[W]hat knowledge or what testimony"[39] can Lacan appeal to in order to verify his assertion about an absence in animal consciousness? Through what means could this claim, made in the negative, conceivably be rationally ascertained?

Once cornered like this, the Lacanian position is fully clarified: One cannot *know* that animals cannot consciously deceive, but we do know that animals cannot articulate to *the (small 'o') other* that they are consciously deceiving—if it is possible at all, it is an act that cannot occur within the symbolic order. Here we have, through Derrida's critique, rendered Lacan more precise: the deception, which Derrida contends could exist, does not transpire via the signifier; the tracks are not covered. Only through articulation—albeit not necessarily through speech—does a psychoanalytic account of 'second degree' deception become possible: one is a subject of a signifier not on account of some hidden capacity that only the individual subject themselves can access; instead, they become a subject of the signifier through capitulation to the intersubjective network of the symbolic order. The self-reflexive deceptive action must undergo some transformation to be decipherable to another—even if the other is not aware they are being deceived, they must still receive *some* transmission for deception to take place.

Through a radical deconstructive procedure, Derrida reminds us to leave an indeterminate epistemological space open for animals and their (speculative) capacity to feign feigning, yet this in no way leads us to conclude that animals are subjects of the signifier. The space can be left open, but it is not filled by animals (or remains yet-to-be-filled); in a word, the epistemological cranny Derrida forces open is *empty*. Derrida's insistence on this empty remainder is significant because differentiating between first-degree deception (feigning; lying in absence of self-consciousness of lying) and second-degree deception (feign feigning; lying with self-consciousness that one is lying) is impossible without a symbolic exchange, and articulating this adds needed precision to Lacan's remarks on animality.

However, on another front, Derrida certainly is correct when he astutely critiques the position that animals remain tethered to the imaginary domain, that they remain "within the snare of the imaginary, thus depriving it of any access to the symbolic."[40] This position, which Derrida attributes to Lacan, would appear to seriously limit the status of animals as subjects—yet, if we return to the texts of Lacan, we see that, while he did at times partially manifest this perspective, it is not entirely stable in his thinking. Animals do partake in the imaginary register, as will be discussed in the subsequent chapter, yet they are in no way limited to this domain in a manner which forecloses human-animal intersubjectivity. Animal subjectivity may be defined by the imaginary, but it can puncture the symbolic via the sign. Lacan clearly acknowledges the position of animals beyond the imaginary, as he writes in Seminar VI:

> Let us return to the hippopotamus. What does this hippopotamus do? . . . he maps out what one can call his territory delimiting it by a series of relays, of points which should sufficiently mark for those who ought to recognise it, namely his fellows, that this is his. This is to show you that I know very well that there are the beginnings of symbolic activity in animals. As you see, in the mammal it is a very specially excremental symbolism. If in short the hippopotamus is found to protect his pasturage with his excrement, we find that the progress realised by man, and in fact this would really not have arisen, if we did not have this particular mediation of language, which comes from we know not where, but it is what causes to intervene here the essential complication, namely that it has led us to this problematic relationship with the object, that for man on his part it is not his pasturage that he protects with shit; therefore it is his shit that he protects as a pledge of the essential pasturage, of the pasturage which is essentially to be determined, and this is the dialectic of what is called anal symbolism.[41]

In this sprawling passage by Lacan on the practice of hippopotamuses to 'symbolically' spread their excrement over land to mark it as their own, we see Lacan concede that animals show the 'beginnings of symbolic activity' and, of course, this activity is not limited to hippos—consider the dog that urinates on an object to 'mark' it as his own. While Lacan never systematically defines the linguistic status of animals, they clearly exceed a purely imaginary state. To explore Lacanian analysis in a manner that exceeds Lacan's own articulation of animals, we must look towards his conception of knowledge, love, and their relation to symbolic processes. There is symbolic activity for the animal—a usage of the sign within the imaginary. Signs function in the field of the imaginary yet can attach to the objects of language for humans—the flap which functions both as sign and signifier (with two corresponding registers, namely that of the imaginary and the symbolic).

Love, Animals, and Knowledge: Can 'The Animal' Love?

Lacan concludes his "Rats in a Maze," and Seminar XX, on this rather cryptic note: "to know what your partner will do is not a proof of love."[42] Here, in a single sentence, we see a thematic composite of the entire seminar; it is a syntactical collision of love, knowledge, and, wedged in the center, the symbolic. What place does language hold in love? And, more importantly, for this chapter's purposes, how does conceiving love and its relation to language elucidate the position of animals?

To begin, language, insofar as it is a demand, is always a demand for love. Lacan says exactly this: "demand, which is initially demand for the satisfaction of a need, turns out to take on a different import as it becomes demand for love."[43]

The modification in demand coincides with the subject becoming a "speaking subject."[44] In short, once the subject's needs are articulated through language (upon their entrance into the symbolic order), they are bound up with a desire that exceeds need—*need* being the instinctually intuited biological processes that, once satisfied, enable the continuation of life. A need can be successfully sated and met through responding to given biological processes: One has the need for food—experienced as hunger—and satisfies that need through the ingestion of food. The need does not linger beyond its fulfillment until its cyclical re-emergence necessarily arises again in the healthy subject.

Once a need becomes articulated through a (linguistic) demand, the need is no longer contained within the biological perpetuation of life (a 'pure' bio-need that can be addressed in its totality); the totality of a demand uttered through language can never be exhausted by the processes which satisfy need. Lacan explicates this precise function of demand articulated through language: "the subject's demand becomes something other than what it explicitly asks for, which is the satisfaction of a need."[45] Consider the following: A pre-lingual newborn baby drinks from their mother's breast (or the bottle) to satisfy the need of hunger. Once the baby drinks, the need is sated. However, when the baby cries for its mother—even if out of hunger-need—the cry does not merely indicate the breast; the cry is a cry for the mother and all that she represents for the baby (love). The issue is compounded when the child actually begins to rely on language: When the baby does enter into the symbolic and asks for 'mama,' the articulation of the need for food, enunciated through speech, is bound to the structure of the signifier and its inherent, self-defining mechanism of substitution. Language, in all its substitutional nature, alienates the child from their demand that must be articulated through the signifier despite its inability to ever name the very thing that is being called for. The subject cannot even "designate themselves" in the "signifying system,"[46] so, naturally, the subject cannot properly, in a totally exhaustive manner, designate the object of demand that transcends bio-need. The utterance of the signifier becomes "a demand for love" for "someone who can be present or absent."[47] Like the cry, the signifier 'mama' contains much more than the mere call for a need to be satisfied—it is a call for love.

Bruce Fink, the prominent Lacanian translator and scholar, writes in his book *Lacan on Love* that,

> All speech is a request or demand for something we are missing, or at least to be heard and recognized as missing something, as lacking in some respect. Ultimately, as Lacan puts it, all speech constitutes a demand for love (38).[48]

What the baby articulates through their cry and their eventual enunciation of 'mama' is the foundation of lack—not the lack of something that can be satisfied like a need, but a persistent, foundational-existential lack that eludes satisfaction. For Lacan, this lack, though it can never be plugged up by any temporal-material-conceptual object, can only be properly met (not satisfied) by love. This demand for love should not be conflated with the diffuse concept of want or desire: albeit demand is tethered to desire, demand is the operation which calls (for love; for recognition; for the thing that symbolically fills the unfillable lack), and desire is the remainder left between the operation (of demand) and its ostensible 'true' object (of need). Desire is the non-necessary dimension of demand abstracted down to its very kernel-core. To return to the babies' call for the mother: the object of need is the breast to satisfy hunger; the demand is for the mother's presence and recognition (her love); and the desire is everything between breast and love—the surplus beyond need that is articulated by demand.

The question that must be submitted, which exceeds the theoretical territory explicitly or directly covered by Lacan himself, is this: What of the dog's bark? If the dog is subject to the superego, and the dog lives among the humans, is its bark exhausted by need? Is the dog's bark not a demand that articulates a lack which exceeds biological processes? Or is it the case that the dog's bark is a limited demand—a demand not for love, but an instinctual desire that remains bound to biological activity and bio-need? For instance, the bark could exceed need in the sense that it is not necessary for the perpetuation of life, but it is still a call for food that is indirectly related to need—an instinct for sustenance that transcends need but is tethered to the biological drive to eat in the name of life itself.

Clearly, the bark does not function as a signifier—this claim can be dismissed outright since there are no combinatory or arbitrary substitutional elements present within the bark-noise (the bark is not understood via phonetic difference corresponding to signifieds)—but it is, nonetheless, clearly a demand articulated through a modality of vocally articulated language (what we may refer to as a sign). A bark, of course, is a communicative act; it is a vessel of (a kind of) language, and this fact cannot be disputed. Keeping this in view, we must discover how this bark potentially acts as a demand in a dimension beyond need. In Seminar VI, Lacan interprets two atypical language-acts that can aid our understanding of the dog's bark: he analyzes the cough and the bark of a dog (issued by a human).

Lacan, in a very thorough and uncharacteristically direct manner, discusses a patient that another early psychoanalyst, Elle Sharpe, analyzed in her writings. While the patient's history and dream-text supply rich analytic material, Lacan in "The Little Cough as a Message" strays from the overt center of the analytic material and instead analyzes the latent symptomatic margins—choosing to delineate the meaning of a cough that the patient issues upon their entrance into the analyst's office. Sharpe, perceptively, does not dismissively cast the cough as a meaningless physical response, but Lacan feels that it must be analyzed with more subtlety, as she seems to recognize the cough contains meaning without diligently interrogating that very meaning. Lacan asserts, like Sharpe, that the cough "is a message";[49] it is an unconscious transmission. While it is not necessary, for our purposes, to index the patient's history or the specificity of the case, it is sufficient to say that, for Lacan, the cough, transpiring right before the analysand walks into where the analysis will take place, is a message of presence—the cough means that "I am here."[50]

Later, the same patient recounts a fantasy in which he "barks like a dog"[51] to avoid detection while engaging in some masturbatory activity or otherwise being someplace he should not be. While this fantasy holds a specific relation to this patient's history, the perceptive insight Lacan comes to is that the bark, while acting as a message of presence, ultimately acts as a message of another's presence—since the analysand is other than a dog. The bark becomes, for the patient, a "signifier . . . of what he is not."[52] Here, we are returned to the sign/signifier distinction since Lacan states in the same seminar that the bark (or any communicative noise an animal utilizes) is a sign "by which the animal presents itself as itself."[53] For the human who issues the bark to elude whoever would find him, there is obviously the double-reflexive, self-erasing movement of the signifier: The human uses the truth, via the bark's immediate 'I am here' (meaning the human is present) in the name of a lie, 'Other than *I* is here' (meaning it is only a dog). The human, who barks behind a closed door, perfectly illustrates the subject of enunciation. When the dog barks, however, the bark remains a truthful sign: 'I am here.' The extractable insight is this: The bark is a sign, a language device, that indicates pure-presence when used by a dog. A bark functions similarly to the operation of the cough, which could be used as a signifier, but could also merely indicate presence, such as announcing your presence in a room you have just entered.

The bark, then, is a communicative sign of presence—but it is still uncertain if this sign of presence is a call for love or remains tethered to bio-need (recognized to fulfill the need for food, which, for the domesticated animal, is dependent on the human to dispense to the animal that makes their presence known). Key to understanding the function of the bark is recognition of the dog's status (along with other domesticated animals) as having a superego in relation to the operation of guilt—and a return to Freud and his thoughts on the development of guilt and the superego will facilitate that very understanding. In *Civilization and Its Discontents*, Freud offers an astute interpretation of guilt's formation in the subject:

> [I]f we ask how a person comes to have a sense of guilt, we arrive at an answer which cannot be disputed: a person feels guilty (devout people would say 'sinful') when he has done something which he knows to be 'bad.' But then we notice how little this answer tells us . . . . [Guilt] can easily be designated as fear of loss of love. If he loses the love of another person upon whom he is dependent, he also ceases to be protected from a variety of dangers.[54]

He explains that this modality of guilt—fearing the loss of love—is predicated on external authority: those who operate according to this underdeveloped guilt "allow themselves to do any bad thing which promises them enjoyment, so long as they are sure that the authority will not know anything about it or cannot blame them for it."[55] Later, Freud explicates the relation between this operation and the superego: this sense of guilt is superseded, in those who undergo full maturation in a psychic sense, by the superego. Once one enters a "higher stage" of "conscience," the "authority is internalized through the establishment of the superego."[56] As

Green succinctly states, authority is "first un-interiorised and then assimilated into the superego"[57]—and this superegoic conscience does not allow for evasion of guilt since there is no longer a distinction between intention (which would remain concealed and internalized) and action (which would be perceptible by external authority); the inner-outer distinction no longer exists, and guilt pervades both domains indiscriminately.

Superegoic guilt accounts for the psychoanalytic fact of guilt detached from a 'bad' action: Due to the internalization of the punitive superego, guilt ceases to be solely a correlate of action—while guilt can certainly still hold a causal relation to action, it can also arise totally estranged from it. Humans (and accordingly all those with a superego) can experience guilt for an (external) act that they did not commit; guilt is dislodged from action and is converted into a free-floating subjective phenomenon on the plane of thought. Guilt's secondary dimension, as that which is unbound to external punishment and even action itself, is exhibited throughout psychoanalytic theory. The prominent psychoanalyst Melanie Klein supplies commentary on this exact idea of unbounded guilt in her essay, "Mourning and Melancholic States." After delineating how a patient who, as a child, phantasizes about a time when "he will be strong, tall and grown up, powerful, rich and potent, and father and mother will have changed into helpless children, or again, in other phantasies, will be very old, weak, poor and rejected," subsequently, much later in life, may be impeded in professional activities "through the guilt to which [the phantasy of triumph] gives rise."[58]

In the same essay, Klein describes a scene from a patient where the analysand's mother is treated in a "patronizing way" by another woman, likely due to the fact that the analysand's brother was being tutored by the woman's son—leaving her to believe that her son (the one who was tutoring the analysand's brother) was more intelligent. Despite this occurring when the analysand was very young, it persisted to her due to "unconscious feelings of guilt. She felt it to be the fulfilment of her own harmful wishes [against her brother]."[59] What can be surmised from these psychoanalytic anecdotes? That guilt exists in the arena of (unconscious) thought (phantasy and death wishes) because of the internalization implanted by the superego. Lacan states, acknowledging the pervasiveness of the superego's procedure, that "something that psychoanalysis has drawn attention to . . . [is] the importance, I would even say the omnipresence, of a sense of guilt."[60] Guilt's "omnipresence" becomes a possibility only through its abstraction from external actions—and there are certainly forms of guilt that go beyond the examples from Klein, guilt that attaches to something that one anticipates that they *might think*, a mode of preemptive guilt.

If we take Lacan seriously and conclude that dogs have a superego (and a capacity for superegoic guilt), then we will come to radical conclusions about their relation to love and the function of the bark. First, though, we must see if we can confirm his claim of the dog's superego: Are dogs capable of the 'higher state' of conscience that Freud attributes to the ego? They are certainly—unequivocally—capable of the lower order of guilt Freud describes. A dog can detect when an action is deemed 'bad' by an external authority. These orders of guilt act as corollaries to the sign/signifier distinction: The human sense of guilt holds an arbitrary relation to external punishment since it is mediated through thought and the superego (like the relation of the human to the signifier); the dog's guilt, conversely, holds an immediate relation to the external punishment (like the relation of the animal to the sign).

When the dog chews on the shoe and subsequently hides herself from the owner—tail between her legs—there is a recognition of 'bad' that will, when discovered by the external authority (in this case, the human), presumably result in a (possibly punitive) judgment of the transgression that has taken place. How is this judgment felt for the dog in question? It is experienced precisely as a (potential) 'loss of love.' The dog acts covertly, attempting to conceal their act, then hides their tail between their legs in shame from a fear of losing love. What does love mean here? It means, in the most immediate and pragmatic sense, loss of care by an-other (there are other, more diffuse and less utilitarian but nonetheless crucial, meanings to human-animal love that will be explored later).

As Freud demonstrated, however, fearing the loss of love does not constitute a superego—if the origin of guilt remains an external authority, imposed from a source estranged from their own conscious, then dogs do not have a true superego in the sense that Freud explicates. That authority must become 'internalized'; the fear itself must be internalized—and the former distinction between intention and execution, thought and action, dissolves. The dog would have to become guilty at the *thought* of chewing on the shoe. Conversely, the guilty thought, severed from an act warranting its arising, accounts for the ubiquity of guilt in the human subject. There appears to be no evidence, theoretical or empirical, that this is the case for the animal: Lacan's declaration of the dog's possession of a superego seems to be an overstatement that exceeds the self-awareness attributable to the species. Lacan comes to this radical (and, as we see, highly contestable) conclusion by observing that, while most animals display an "immediate indifference that most animals show towards remainders, towards the corpses of their fellows once they have become corpses,"[61] dogs are an exception in the sense that they exhibit "attachment to a dead person."[62] From this, Lacan determines that though dogs do not have an "unconscious," they do have a "superego, namely that something has come into play which allows there to be something of the order of a certain delineation of signifying articulation."[63]

The superegoic operation that Lacan attributes to dogs is clearly symbolic—and the signifier (or, more accurately, sign) that comes 'into play' for the dog, that the dog recognizes through attachment rather than the expected animal 'indifference,' is precisely the corpse (presumably here of the owner). It is questionable, though, that the superego—in the technical sense deployed by Freud—is the 'something' that permits this signifying articulation to occur; it is apparent, rather, that Lacan's conception of the dog's recognition of the articulation made by the corpse aligns with Freud's pre-internalized primary guilt: The dog perceives the corpse's operation as a sign which articulates a loss of love—the corpse is, for the dog, the very sign of a loss of love that is grieved, in some manner, and is tethered to the function of guilt and its relation to the external authority. This is the case, of course, because the corpse is only recognized as a loss of love if the one who has died could also potentially be a source of guilt: The dog only grieves the body for which a guilty experience, if they engaged in an act that would be judged as 'bad,' were possible.

The fact that dogs experience a pre-superegoic form of guilt reliant on the other's judgment does not mean we abandon dogs' relation to love: The modality of guilt that dogs are susceptible to places them, clearly, within a dimension of love. Grief and guilt (particularly prior to the proper formation of the superego) are found to be inextricably formed around a central nexus of love—both are concerned with one's status as 'loved' (in the non-linguistic sense) by one who represents a source of love. To return to the initial line of thought: What of the dog's bark? Is the dog's bark (which we have defined as a sign of presence) a demand for love which operates like the baby's utterance for their mother ('mama')? Through the procedure of guilt—knowing that the dog's knowledge of 'bad' (as judged by the external authority) coincides with a fear of loss of love—we can confirm dog's operate in the domain of eros, and this procedure informs us of the bark: If guilt is the fear of loss of love, the bark holds an obverse function; the dog's bark is a demand in the register of love—a bark, or at least a certain modality of bark, a particular tenor of bark, is a call for love engendered via a vocal reminder of presence. *The dog's bark is a sign of presence calling for love.*

In *Lacan on Love*, Fink writes that animals are only capable of "attachment" rather than what we would call proper human love. His example to illustrate this point is pertinent to our line of thought:

> [W]e might talk about certain forms of attachment as related to love. But they might also be characterized as mere liking that has grown out of habit, out of being thrown together . . . . We can wonder, for example, whether a bear cub—which has clearly been attached to its mother for about two years of its life . . . experiences the effects of separation from a loved one the way human beings do . . . . If we are to not call what the bear experiences "love," are we then claiming that love requires the kind of memory that only human beings have, the kind of memory that is linguistically structured for the most part, allowing us to conjure up thoughts and images and feelings related to the beloved simply be repeating his or her name? Is what we are calling love, then, characteristic of human beings alone?[64]

Fink makes a necessary intervention here, a puncture in the discourse on love—love cannot merely be reduced to attachment "grown out of habit"—reducing the radical, inexhaustible flow of love to preferential attachment to an-other is not a coherent articulation of love. Instead, Fink indirectly imparts the Lacanian limit of love: a linguistic structure that designates, in memory, the other as loved and brings with it pain. Fink reminds us that pain is always the alternate of love, and that it exists only through the temporary submergence entailed by painful loss (one should detect here a similar topographical relation in a different dimension: that of desire and its corresponding lack, the perpetual cavity that activates desire).

Fink's contention may certainly be accurate—love should not be reduced to emotionally-invested attachment; love does exceed attachment and subsists on a grounding of pain (if lost or even at the conception of loss itself). But our designation of dog-love *does* subsist on pain (the pain of guilt) and remains exempt from a formal linguistic structure—there is a binding of love and loss for the dog. And, while one could attempt to granularly distinguish between the dog-love and human-love, we find here that the sign (the sign of the other—the owner—and the bark) mediates access to the exact love Fink describes.

While what exactly 'love' is remains opaque and will be returned to in later chapters, we can now refer again to Lacan's concluding line in "The Rats in the Maze": "to know what your partner will do is not a proof of love."[65] Obviously, in the most immediate sense, this refers to behaviorism and the rats: The behavioral researchers have knowledge of what the rat within the maze will do; they know that the rat will hit the flap. Yet, according to Lacan, this is not love—as he says, the researchers chose rats because "one can easily make a unit of it"[66] and claims that the researchers actually had a "hatred" for the rats. These statements appear confounding—unless, that is, we return to the definition of guilt lost love by Freud and Fink's statements on demand and love, where we find that love is predicated on presence, and this grants us an initial insight: If the other's presence is love, and the other's absence spurs the fear of loss of love (related to the impulse of guilt and grief), then knowing what the other "will do"—a full epistemological assimilation of the other's presence—must be the highest degree of love.

Lacan makes it clear that love is, in some foundational way, contingent on presence and, concurrently, irreducible to presence: The recognition of the other's presence, knowledge of the other, is not love. In short, the dog's bark, when acknowledged by the human, does not indicate love. The demand for love is not met—it is never entirely satisfied in its totality—merely by presence or knowledge of presence. There is a confrontation that exceeds knowledge and the symbolic, which occurs within the register of the Real and the imaginary, where true love takes place. In terms of the symbolic, we can say this: The dog can love, and our evidence is found in their guilt and the function of their bark. While we cannot speak of *the animal* as this amorphous, monolithic uni-group, we also should not hastily consider dogs a complete and utter aberration of animality. If the dog can love, then love is an arena that is not totally monopolized by the human—the category of human and animals, while necessary and useful, shifts upon this realization; the human is not the only being who loves.

Notes

1 Jacques Lacan, *The Ethics of Psychoanalysis: The Seminar of Jacques Lacan, Book VII*, ed. Jacques-Alain Miller, trans. Dennis Porter (New York: W. W. Norton & Company, 1992), 45.
2 Jacques Lacan, *Desire and Its Interpretation: The Seminar of Jacques Lacan, Book VI*, ed. Jacques-Alain Miller, trans. Bruce Fink (Cambridge: Polity Press, 2019), 139.

3 Noam Chomsky, review of *Verbal Behavior*, by B. F. Skinner, *Language* 35, no. 1 (1959): 26–58.
4 Sigmund Freud, *An Outline of Psycho-Analysis*, trans. James Strachey (New York: W. W. Norton & Company, 1969), 14.
5 Jacques Lacan, *The Formations of the Unconscious: The Seminar of Jacques Lacan, Book V*, ed. Jacques-Alain Miller, trans. Russell Grigg (Cambridge: Polity Press, 2017), 325.
6 Hub Zwart, "Conditioned Reflexes and the Symbolic Order: A Lacanian Assessment of Ivan Pavlov's Experimental Practice," *Vestigia: The Journal of the International Network of Psychotherapeutic Practice* (2018): 59.
7 Lacan, *Formations of the Unconscious*, 325.
8 Jacques Lacan, *On Feminine Sexuality, the Limits of Love and Knowledge: The Seminar of Jacques Lacan, Book XX, Encore*, ed. Jacques-Alain Miller, trans. Bruce Fink (New York: W. W. Norton & Company, 1998), 141.
9 Lacan, *Desire and Its Interpretation*, 13.
10 Jacques Lacan, *Écrits*, trans. Bruce Fink (New York: W. W. Norton & Company, 2006), 245–246.
11 Lacan, *Écrits*, 245.
12 Lacan, *Écrits*, 246.
13 Lacan, *Écrits*, 13.
14 Lacan, *Desire and Its Interpretation*, 139.
15 Lacan, *Desire and Its Interpretation*, 76.
16 Lacan, *Desire and Its Interpretation*, 16.
17 Lacan, *Écrits*, 713.
18 Lacan, *Ethics of Psychoanalysis*, 45.
19 Sean Meighoo, "Human Language, Animal Code, and the Question of Beeing," *Humanimalia* 8, no. 2 (2017): 39.
20 Meighoo, "Human Language, Animal Code, and the Question of Beeing," 39.
21 Meighoo, "Human Language, Animal Code, and the Question of Beeing," 39.
22 Peter Buse, "The Dog and the Parakeet: Lacan Among the Animals," *Angelaki: Journal of Theoretical Humanities* 22, no. 4 (2017): 24.
23 Jacques Derrida, *The Animal That Therefore I Am*, ed. Marie-Louise Mallet, trans. David Wills (New York: Fordham University Press, 2008), 78.
24 See Teddy Duncan, Jr., *Interpreting Meat: Theorizing the Commodification and Consumption of Animals* (Jefferson, NC: McFarland, 2024).
25 Freud, *An Outline of Psycho-Analysis*, 19.
26 Jacques Lacan, *The Seminar of Jacques Lacan, Book II: The Ego in Freud's Theory and in the Technique of Psychoanalysis*, ed. Jacques-Alain Miller, trans. Sylvana Tomaselli (New York: W. W. Norton & Company, 1991), 84.
27 Lacan, *Écrits*, 683.
28 Lacan, *Écrits*, 683.
29 Lacan, *Desire and Its Interpretation*, 89.
30 Lacan, *Four Fundamental Concepts*, 139.
31 Lacan, *Desire and Its Interpretation.*
32 Sigmund Freud, *Jokes and Their Relation to the Unconscious*, trans. James Strachey (New York: W. W. Norton & Company, 1989), 137–138.
33 Freud, *Jokes and Their Relation to the Unconscious*, 138.
34 Derrida, *The Animal That Therefore I Am*, 133.
35 Derrida, *The Animal That Therefore I Am*, 133.
36 Derrida, *The Animal That Therefore I Am*, 135.
37 Derrida, *The Animal That Therefore I Am*, 135.
38 Derrida, *The Animal That Therefore I Am*, 128.
39 Derrida, *The Animal That Therefore I Am*, 133.
40 Derrida, *The Animal That Therefore I Am*, 120.

41 Lacan, *Desire and Its Interpretation*, 106.
42 Lacan, *Encore*, 146.
43 Lacan, *Desire and Its Interpretation*, 375.
44 Lacan, *Desire and Its Interpretation*, 375.
45 Lacan, *Desire and Its Interpretation*, 371.
46 Lacan, *Desire and Its Interpretation*, 367.
47 Lacan, *Desire and Its Interpretation*, 395.
48 Bruce Fink, *Lacan on Love: An Exploration of Lacan's Seminar VIII, Transference* (Cambridge: Polity Press, 2016), 38.
49 Lacan, *Desire and Its Interpretation*, 149.
50 Lacan, *Desire and Its Interpretation*, 150.
51 Lacan, *Desire and Its Interpretation*, 161.
52 Lacan, *Desire and Its Interpretation*, 163.
53 Lacan, *Desire and Its Interpretation*, 164.
54 Sigmund Freud, *Civilization and Its Discontents*, trans. James Strachey (New York: W. W. Norton & Company, 1961), 84–85.
55 Freud, *Civilization and Its Discontents*, 86.
56 Freud, *Civilization and Its Discontents*, 86.
57 André Green, *On the Destruction and Death Drives*, trans. Steven Jaron, ed. Howard B. Levine (London: Phoenix Publishing House, 2023), 88.
58 Melanie Klein, "Mourning and Its Relation to Manic-Depressive States," in *Selected Melanie Klein*, ed. Juliet Mitchell (New York: Simon and Schuster, 1987), 154.
59 Klein, "Mourning and Its Relation to Manic-Depressive States," 159.
60 Lacan, *Ethics of Psychoanalysis*, 3.
61 Lacan, *Desire and Its Interpretation*, 89.
62 Lacan, *Desire and Its Interpretation*, 89.
63 Lacan, *Desire and Its Interpretation*, 89.
64 Bruce Fink, *Lacan on Love: An Exploration of Lacan's Seminar VIII, Transference* (Cambridge: Polity Press, 2016), 110.
65 Lacan, *Encore*, 146.
66 Lacan, *Encore*, 146.

Chapter 2

Lacan's Pigeons

Animals in the Imaginary Register

The most endemic, and trite, criticisms of Lacan relate to his ostensibly unwarranted primacy of the signifier—and the symbolic register—above all; some banal thinkers accuse Lacan of reducing everything to language, claiming that he engaged in a thoughtless, and hyper-idealist, post-structuralist project of semantic-based nihilistic relativism. According to these theoreticians, for Lacan, everything is language. Meaning truth, along with empirical-veridical reality, remains utterly outside the bounds of his theoretical grasp. There is only language—and all else that supposedly exceeds language, all that appears to be supra-lingual, is actually latently linguistically constructed. Lacan even appears to confirm this misapprehension of his work, insisting that psychoanalytic concepts only "take on their full meaning when oriented in a field of language and ordered in relation to the function of speech."[1] At this point, we neatly arrive at the criticisms issued, implicitly and sometimes even explicitly, by animal studies against Lacanian thought: There is not adequate space allotted for the animal in Lacanian theory; animals, due to being precluded from the symbolic, are relegated to the ineffable dimension of the Real or the purely illusory-optical register of the imaginary.

As we saw in the previous chapter, animals are not totally outside the system of language—the animal may not have access to the symbolic (the law of the signifier), but they have the sign, which erects a certain intelligibility in the world and the possibility of cross-species (animal-to-human) intersubjectivity. Additionally, as numerous Lacanians have insisted before, the imaginary is not synonymous with 'the illusory.' Lacan consistently asserts throughout his work that "the imaginary is not an illusion."[2] Operating within the specular dimension of the imaginary does not somehow render a given experience less substantive, reduce its ontological density, or attenuate it in any meaningful way. Camille Paglia succinctly explicates, while referring to ancient human civilizations, that "[w]ords are not the only measure of mental development."[3] We can easily ascertain how Paglia's linguistic anti-determinism translates to animals: The symbolic is not the "only measure" of subjectivity. Imaginary mechanisms also indicate a subjectivity—albeit a subjectivity more alien to the human whose phenomenal reality is mediated (or, in the Lacanian-psychoanalytic lexicon, castrated) by the symbolic. Despite a certain incomprehension of the imaginary register for humans (engendered by the

DOI: 10.4324/9781003635383-4

intervention of the signifier and its primacy in our existence—in our understanding of being; this 'incomprehension' can be understood as a lack of immediacy), Lacan indubitably established the relation between animals and the scopic field: If the symbolic (language dictated by the signifier) is the primary mediating domain of humanity, then the imaginary (the specular dimension of identifications and recognition) is the domain of animality. As Lacan writes, "[o]nly the subject—the human subject, the subject of the desires that is the essence of man—is not, unlike the animal, entirely caught up in this imaginary capture."[4] The human subject is instead "caught up" in a symbolic capture. An unresolved, *gnawing* question remains: What does it mean to be an animal subject within the imaginary register?

This orientation—towards a Lacanian view of animal subjectivity in the imaginary—is necessarily modulated and qualified by the critics of Lacan who posit that his view of language obscures non-linguistic functions, that his primacy of the signifier dilutes non-symbolic activities. Derrida clearly espouses this view, writing (in the same essay mentioned in the preceding chapter) that Lacan restricts the domain of symbolic activity to humans and leaves animals without "any access to the symbolic."[5] While, as I will delineate, it is certainly not true that Lacan limits his analysis to the symbolic (it is well known that Lacan's later seminars incorporate, more and more, the Real and jouissance)—and it is doubly false that he ever asserts that there is nothing but language—Lacan has isolated the symbolic, the signifier's structure, to be the originary emergent-site of (human) subjectivity. Lacan may not assert that everything is language or limit his analysis to the symbolic and human language, but he did attempt to render (human) subjectivity and the symbolic co-concomitant, if not synonymous. To establish a theoretical model of a different kind of subjectivity, an animal subjectivity that relies on imaginary formations (along with the sign), we must concurrently contend with Lacan's views on the imaginary and subjectivity in general.

The Pigeon, the Monkey, and the Mirror Stage: Imaginary Subjectivity

Lacan's seminal text on the mirror stage, "The Mirror Stage as Formative of the *I* Function as Revealed in Psychoanalytic Experience," provides a revolutionary, explicit entry-point into the imaginary register and its relation to animality. The essay primarily centers on experiential human self-unity precipitated by the baby seeing themselves in the mirror—and, later on, being told by an-other, *that's you*—the text informs us that the saga of the ego, its developmental procedure, unfurling from the babies' preceding state of fractured disjuncture, of limitless non-cohesion, is terminated by the synthesis (an image of static, pre-defined unity) offered by the mirror's self-reflective image. Ego begins as an external image of oneself—in the literal sense of an optical-visual representation of oneself—gazing back. In order to arrive at this profound observation on the operation of the mirror-image, which tells us so much about human ego-formation, Lacan digressively passes through animality.

On the very first page of the essay, Lacan delineates the function of the mirror for the human and the monkey:

> the human child, at an age when he is for a short while, but for a while nevertheless, outdone by the chimpanzee in instrumental intelligence, can already recognize his own image as such in a mirror . . . this act, far from exhausting itself, as in the case of a monkey, in eventually acquired control over the uselessness of the image, immediately gives rise in a child to a series of gestures in which he playfully experiences the relationship between the movements made in the image and the reflected environment, and between this virtual complex and the reality it duplicates, namely, the child's own body.[6]

The child, who Lacan notes is fleetingly surpassed by the chimpanzee in terms of motor-functional ability and corporeal control, self-recognizes themself in the mirror despite their premature functional state, and this proffers them a unified stratification of self—from head to toes—activated by the specular image of (imaginary) unity. Prior to the baby gaining the physical and cognitive capacity for motor-functional unity (which the monkey gains much more quickly), they recognize themselves in the mirror—and for Lacan, this recognition initiates the child into self-hood. The mirror stage marks the movement from a disjointed, indistinct mass of universality (egolessness) to an enclosed bodily form that coheres, delimits, and unifies in a singular, indivisible image of self (ego-formation). As critical animal studies scholar Hub Zwart succinctly comments on Lacan's text: "It is only when we begin to recognize ourselves in a mirror that we manage to see ourselves as a unity, a whole."[7] Before the mirror stage, there is no united self for the infant, only a dispersed non-self indistinguishable from the rest of the encountered universe.

It is critical that Lacan begins with bio-physiological species-based difference. This rhetorical move illustrates the singular significance of the imaginary ego-development for the child; the ego-formation, in the child's progression towards adulthood, precedes even basic psychomotor activity—what Lacan calls 'anatomical incompleteness.' Lacan inserts another crucial distinction: The mirror image is 'exhausted for the monkey, but the image remains presumably inexhaustible for the human-child who engages in a series of 'playful gestures.' What does this mean for the monkey and their relation to the function of the mirror? The monkey's self-reflective image, according to Lacan, does not lead to the same binding fascination with specularity that it holds for the human baby—Lacan is not only identifying a physical difference between monkeys and humans, but he is also, far more radically, attempting to detect the inaugural moment that splits animality and humanity into egolessness and ego-centricism. Unlike the baby, for the monkey there is no mirror stage and hence no united ego.

However, this claim should be qualified and necessarily revised: While Lacan is correct that monkeys do not engage in spontaneous self-recognition upon seeing their image in the mirror (unlike human-babies, dolphins, or great apes), new research has emerged (as it is apt to do over a period of nearly a century) demonstrating that certain sub-species of monkeys, specifically the rhesus monkey (among other species such as dolphins), can be trained to recognize themselves in the mirror and engage in gestures similar to those Lacan solely attributes to the human-child. After a period of habituating young monkeys to mirrors through 30-minute exposure periods, using a "mirror-facing head-fixation chair," and afterwards using "visual-proprioceptive"[8] training relying on laser pointers and food rewards, beginning with shining the light on points of their bodies the monkeys could see, then gradually moving to points that only could be seen through the virtual self-image of the mirror (for instance, the forehead), researchers concluded that the monkey recognized themselves in the mirror (since the monkeys reached towards spots only visible via the mirror). The trained monkeys even exhibited "spontaneous mirror-induced self-directed behaviors"[9] that included self-examination of genitals by using the mirror-image. These same monkeys, which Lacan dismissed as cognitively and psychically unequipped with contending with the inexhaustibility of the mirror-image, have demonstrated "bodily self-consciousness"[10]—a distance, an irrevocable gap between self and other, which encloses the self in a specular (imaginary) unity and coalesces the fragmentation of the body into a coherent totality. Specularity, then, is not only available to the human-baby but the thoroughly trained monkey as well.

Monkeys are not the only reference to animality in Lacan's essay dealing with scopic properties and the imaginary field—equally conspicuous is the mention of pigeons and their reproductive practices:

> it is a necessary condition for the maturation of the gonad of the female pigeon that it should see another member of its species, of either sex; so sufficient in itself is this condition that the desired effect may be obtained merely by placing the individual within reach of the field of reflection of a mirror.[11]

According to Lacan, in order for the female pigeon to gain gonadic maturation to reproduce, they must see themselves in another—another externalized and visually available version of themselves, not on the individual level, but on the species level (it is not that they must see themselves, instead they must see a variant of themselves—here there is not self-identification, but rather species identification). Lacan also links this to the activities of locusts:

> Similarly, in the case of the migratory locust, the transition within a generation from the solitary to the gregarious form can be obtained by exposing the individual, at a certain stage, to the exclusively visual action of a similar image.[12]

In both instances, Lacan detects the imaginary function of mimicry in the realm of animality and deploys these examples to situate the *image* within biological phenomenon—as Peter Buse explains, "Lacan grants to the animal a specular function, which is to say, a relation to its *semblable*, or mirror-image."[13] The visual field, which appears superfluous in the development of an organism, instead appears to be vitally indispensable to maturation. While a simple, and what some may find to be very clever, objection to Lacan's notions is some variant of the following: *What of the congenitally blind child? Do they not gain a sense of self, instead operating in a free-floating umwelt-world without distinction between self and other?* The answer here is the perception-consciousness system which exceeds visuality but can regardless be referred to as *image*.

The distinction here, between the procedure of gonad development in pigeons and the mimicry of the locusts versus the function of the mirror for human-babies and monkeys, should be clear: For the monkey and baby, the mirror acts as a resounding designation of (non-linguistic) 'I'—the self-referential specular image binds the ego and implants the bounds of that ego-self (which, for the human baby, will later be the linguistic 'I' function) in consciousness. The pigeons and locusts, however, engage in pure mimicry—while there is a degree of self-image (the pigeon must see a pigeon; the locust must see something locust-like), pigeons and locusts are assimilating an external image that they then *take on* the attributes of. The pigeon and locust are not identifying themselves with a self-referential image on the visual plane and thereby establishing the bounds of their self-hood (establishing an ego); for the pigeon and the locust, there is no bodily self-consciousness as there is for the monkey and the baby. A pigeon integrates an external image rather than integrating an image that they take to be internal—the distinction between self and other remains permeable and consciously non-existent, although biologically present as a unit in opposition to the world (which explains why one fights, reproduces, and consumes for oneself rather than another—there is no ambiguity on the biological level in terms of instincts and needs of where the self ends and begins, though this may be distinct from the conscious level). Despite these differences—the human, monkey, pigeon, and the locust—are all operating in the imaginary register, simply occupying different tenors of the scopic function.

Visuality does not exhaust the imaginary plane—it is the entire sensory network that engenders identifications. The sensory network is precisely where many are most intimately familiar with the phenomenological division of animality and humanity: We are told they access certain senses (sight, smell) in ways we simply cannot. Why do these enhanced sensory abilities exist across much of animality? Because the senses are the nexus of their subjectivity. Marc Bekoff and Jessica Pierce write that animal olfaction (only one facet of an animal's sensory network) is a biological instrument for identification and kin-recognition for many animals: "many animals recognize kin through an incredibly nuanced sense of smell, and kin smell different from nonkin. Siblings who are reared in the same nest [in the case of birds] acquire one another's odor, and this facilitates kin recognition."[14] Vision, then, is only one sense among many constitutive of an animal's imaginary plane, with the olfactory system being another mode through which animals register identifications: Images are not restricted to the visual field.

Since animals only have access to the sign, instead of the full register of the symbolic, we can ascertain that animal subjectivity is mediated by the imaginary, rather than the symbolic. They are not, as some imprecisely claim, totally chained to the Real. Further, being mediated by the imaginary, rather than the human-symbolic, does not maintain an irrevocable division between animality and humanity—since, as we have seen, the animal has the sign that exceeds the imaginary and permits porousness in the domestic scene—a human-animal intersubjectivity. Let us begin here: What can be known about animal subjectivity in the register of the imaginary? Does it remain inaccessibly opaque—forever at an incomprehensible distance? According to Lacan, the imaginary, specifically the event of the mirror stage, holds a central place in engendering (human) ego-subjectivity:

> the function of the mirror stage . . . is to establish a relationship between an organism and its reality . . . the mirror stage is a drama whose internal pressure pushes precipitously from insufficiency to anticipation—and, for the subject caught up in the lure of spatial identification, turns out fantasies that proceed from a fragmented image of the body to what I will call an 'orthopedic' form of its totality—and to the finally donned armor of an alienating identity that will mark his entire mental development with its rigid structure.[15]

We see here that the specular drive governs the "alienating identity" (the image-of-oneself-severed-from-oneself) engendered by the mirror-image. This "spatial identification" with a "totality" marks the establishment of the ego—the very fantasy-bounds of the individual—and spurs the "relationship between an organism and its reality." In other words, for the human, self-recognition of the mirror-image is the origin of a cohesive, if phantasmic, imaginary subjectivity. The mirror births a relation between an internality and an externality—whereas before the mirror, there is no inner-outer distinction, only a continuity of *in-out, me-all.*

If the mirror stage holds such a pivotal status—acting as a privileged, indispensable juncture—in the development of human subjectivity and ego-formation, why would the imaginary not lead us to insights into animal subjectivity? This inquiry is particularly pertinent when some animals (like, as we have seen, the monkey) cannot be precluded from the same self-recognition a human infant experiences. In terms of the monkey, the dolphin, and the ape—those animals who, to varying degrees and through diverging means, can confer their corporeal image a designation of non-linguistic 'self' (those who experience self-identification)—the imaginary clearly introduces an ego-formation, however limited or tethered to instinctual processes. The monkey who employs the mirror-image to groom their genitals clearly participates in a discernment between *self and other, in-and-out, all-and-me*—there is a bodily-spatial horizon that demarcates the monkey's subjectivity. The monkey articulates, visually, that there is no 'me' beyond this image that is, somehow, in a manner exceeding monkey comprehension, representative of me-ness.

However, as Clive Wynne and Monique Udell clarify, "Most other species tested [other than monkeys, dolphins, and gorillas], including fish, dogs, cats, and parrots, typically react to themselves in the mirror (if at all) as if their reflection were another animal."[16] Simply, most animals do not have bodily self-awareness. For the animal who does not experience bodily self-recognition (and the pre-mirror stage human baby), the body is auto-immanence: without any conceptions of anything, one defecates, urinates, stares, and runs—all this occurs through the immediate relation one takes with one's own body. In Heideggerian language, the infant and animal are "thrown" into "Being-in-the-world"[17]—crucially, though, this occurs supposedly in the absence of the reflexive self-consciousness that Dasein abides in. A mirror-image, for an animal that does not operate beyond this realm of auto-immanence, should be nothing more than a non-substantive, severed bit of meaninglessness; the mirror-image should be an optical non-event that dissolves in flatness (an animal falsely realizing that another poor animal—the image of themselves misrecognized as another—is trapped in a rectangular prison is certainly distinct from realizing that the image is oneself). However, the monkey, like the baby, is a persistent, crucial reminder that subjectivity is not totalized by the adult human subject—interiority is irreducible to a binary between bodily auto-immanence of the non-mirror stage animal and the bodily self-distance ("alienating armor") that the symbolic register affords the human subject.

The next move that Lacan emphasizes in the development of a human child, the essential movement from the imaginary to the symbolic register where the human enters into the symbolic universe through language and enacted discourse, does not take place in animals. Animals participate, unequivocally, in the imaginary arena of identifications and specular functions. Zwart explains that while humans irrevocably penetrate the symbolic network, entering into a linguistically mediated reality, animals "dwell in a different 'imaginary' world, dominated by images."[18] Lacan's example of the Locusts and Pigeons, along with our contemporary knowledge of the monkey, inform us that animals engage in the imaginary register across a variable species-based spectrum. For the Locusts and Pigeons, there is some recognition of *like-me*; for the monkey, dolphin, elephant, and ape, there is recognition of pre-lingual, image-constituted, *me.* How do we reconcile this with the rest of our knowledge of animals? For those animals who do recognize themselves in the mirror, we must situate them in a subjective-cognitive space of tentative, partial egoness. There is a pre-lingual self-presence (for the monkey, dolphin, elephant, ape) that unites the multiplicity of bodily auto-immanence. For those animals who do not transcend that corporeal fragmentation, we can still engage in an analysis of their subjectivity on the visual-scopic (imaginary) plane they operate in.

Consider, again, the domesticated house cat. How do they encounter the world in terms of phenomenological interiority? While there may be some 'signs' the cat accesses (as defined in the preceding chapter, such as the 'flap' for the rat in the maze), we can assume that the cat holds a primarily visual-sensory (audio-visual-tactile) relation to the world: the Real is mediated not through the symbolic, but instead through the imaginary—yet this imaginary has not developed into a totalized ego-hood. Take this common scene: The cat, lying on their stomach, swings their tail and is suddenly startled by its presence, and upon being startled, begins to pounce on their own tail as if it were an object detached from themselves—the tail is not recognized as a bodily-part of the 'I'-whole, but rather as an externalized thing. How is this possible, when the same cat will later clean their tail, implicitly designating it as part of a pre-lingual 'me'? This is because the cat occupies an imaginary domain analogous to the pre-mirror stage baby: Lacan describes the pre-mirror stage baby as existing in a "fragmented body" that transitions into an " 'orthopedic' form of its totality"[19] (due to identification with the mirror-image). The cat's subjectivity resides in this pre-specular condition of fragmentation—their own tail can be mis-recognized as an external-object because the cat-body remains a non-unified multiplicity of parts and domains.

However, paradoxically, despite the cat (and other pre-specular animals) being non-totalized in a unified corporeal delineation, they are not 'alienated' from themselves. Lacan describes the identification with the mirror image that the baby experiences as the "donned armor of an alienating identity that will mark his entire mental development with its rigid structure."[20] The pre-lingual specular image 'I' that the human baby adopts is *forever alienating*—there always remains a foundational discordance between this imaginary image "donned" and the self-subject it designates and attempts to seamlessly unify. Alienation occurs due to *identification*, which immediately permits a gap between image and self (the unified image does not correspond to the experiential multiplicity of subjectivity)—for the cat, therefore, they remain un-alienated. In a sense, mirror image engenders a unification, resulting in a non-union that the pre-specular subject never passes through, from auto-immanence (pre-specular multiplicity) to alienating identification (specular unification). A cat assaults their tail precisely because they are not alienated from their body—the cat knows the body in a modality of immediacy (in absence of total-unity) that the human (post mirror stage) could never experience. The cat's body may not be singular, but it does possess a self.

The Imaginary, the Pre-Specular, and the Gaze: What Is Seen in the Animal Look?

The animal gaze is oftentimes taken to be an utterly inexplicable site of non-access—the look of an animal is assumed to be hermeneutically sealed off, entirely uninterpretable. Derrida's comments on the "bottomless"[21] and "unreadable"[22] animal gaze are often cited on this point to demonstrate its "inexhaustible" nature. To Derrida, the animal gaze is not empty, devoid of autonomous subjectivity (as some suppose); it is instead precisely the obverse: The animal gaze is totally, overwhelmingly full of an impenetrable meaning and self-hood. How could one begin to overcome this inscrutable boundary that the animal gaze represents? Should this not be performed in the register of scientism and ceded to the proper domain of the Zoologist or the Ethologist?

Philip Armstrong, in his chapter "The Gaze of Animals," describes the history of theorizing on animals' gazes. He writes that "[t]he human experience of discomfiture before the gaze of other animals has a long genealogy."[23] He details the movement from pre-modernity when "the eyes of animals were thought to emit a physical force, an irradiation with the power to transfix or infect those who encountered it"[24] to modernity and the advent of science, where the animal gaze is submitted to "geometrical theories of vision" and consequently undermines the "visual agency"[25] of animals. Any animal can see, but only the human comprehends the geometric-mathematical substance of sight: True optical experience is "reduced to a series of two-dimensional planes"[26]—the earlier pre-modern discomfort with the animal gaze is surmounted through a purely scientific understanding of the optical function. Armstrong later details the emerging postmodern perception in the late 20th century that again rendered the gaze of animals "challenging or even menacing"[27] through the manner in which the insistent look signifies "a crisis in the psycho-social foundations of contemporary urban life."[28] The gaze of animality again takes on its pre-modern manifestation as that which cannot be subdued to human forces—it eludes the mathematical gaze of scientism, and there is an undomesticated, *feral* surplus that remains: a remainder of animality that does not auto-submit to the human optical function which mathematizes and condenses.

Armstrong, for a fleeting moment (a page), discusses Freud's writing on animals, and accuses him—and implicitly the entire field of psychoanalysis—of being emblematic of the "effacement of the animal gaze"[29] perpetrated by modern science. He explains that "real animals are interpreted by Freud as representations of unconscious fears and desires . . . Freudian theory epitomizes the transposition . . . of animality into fantasy, myth, dream and fiction, and the associated eclipse of the animal gaze."[30] Armstrong is not the only one who charges psychoanalysis with a reductive transposition of animals into fantasy, myth, and unconscious processes—scholar Nicholas Ray also finds that, while "animals seem to be virtually everywhere"[31] in Freud's famous case studies, "he regards them as dissimulations, as manifest representations standing in for, and disguising, something else."[32] Ray and Armstrong rely on similar examples—Little Hans' phobic view of horses, which Freud transposes for the fear of the parental figure,[33] and Wolfman's dream of wolves staring at him, which Freud also submits to Oedipalization, claiming that the wolves in the dream are "representations of the boy's father"[34]—to display the inability of psychoanalysis to contend with animality.

Both find that psychoanalysis, and specifically Freud, dismiss the reality of animality—and for Armstrong this dismissal immediately relates to psychoanalysis's treatment of the animal gaze. The animal gaze, according to this critique of psychoanalysis, is rendered as a pure-specular reflection of the unconscious desires of a given human who encounters the gaze; the gaze is voided of any self-content (interiority on behalf of the animal) and instead is recapitulated as a phantasmic mirror of the human's psychoanalytic condition. The gaze becomes refracted and intelligible only through the reciprocal gaze of humanity. This contention is not unfounded—it is substantiated by the clinical literature itself: psychoanalysis does frequently reduce the animal to a mere representative object of the human unconscious. To provide an emblematic example: Melanie Klein, in her article "Mourning and Its Relation to Manic-Depressive States," recounts the dream of an analysand in which a bull is a central figure. Klein describes the following dream:

> He saw a bull lying in a farmyard. It was not quite dead, and looked very uncanny and dangerous. He was standing on one side of the bull, his mother on the

> other. He escaped into a house, feeling that he was leaving his mother behind in danger and that he should not do so; but he vaguely hoped that she would get away.[35]

Notably, as Freud stipulates in his *Interpretation of Dreams*, the bull material emerges from an actual recent encounter with a bull (corresponding to the basic dream-principle of material being derived from recent experiences, normally the span of time since one last slept). The analysand had "lately" seen an "actual bull on a friend's farm" and says that it looked "ghastly" and had "urgently advised" his friend to keep the bull under control.[36] What interpretation does Klein assign to this appearance of the bull? For Klein, the bull-dream is "a representation of the dangers by which he felt threatened internally"[37] and related to the imminent death of the analysand's mother that "meant to him her being destroyed by the bull inside him."[38] Although the interpretation by Klein is cast in a peculiar form due to object-relations theory, we see here that the materiality and literalness of the bull is negated in the name of the bull's internal representative fantasy-function: the animal becomes a feature of the unconscious and loses its physical being—and this reduction is indicative of the psychoanalytic approach to animality that both Ray and Armstrong are critical of. Fear—brought about by the encounter with the bull's radically alterior animality—is entirely annulled: The animal is negated in the name of the subjective.

While Ray and Armstrong construct compelling arguments (corroborated by various psychoanalytic approaches), including Kleinian analysis, and indeed present cogent polemics against a kind of psychoanalytic anthropocentric reductivism (despite the obvious fact that a *representation* of an animal and the *physio-empirical* animal itself should be carefully demarcated), we do not need to follow them in the conventional (quite 'postmodern') dispensation of psychoanalysis. Armstrong writes at the end of his chapter that "In bringing together philosophy, the arts, and the sciences, perhaps our new theories about animals—our new ways of 'gazing upon' them—will allow us to learn from animals as well as about them."[39] I would note that psychoanalysis, alongside these other fields (since it is clear psychoanalysis fits neatly neither into the category of science nor philosophy), can make a considerable contribution to this multi-disciplinary approach: We should take Armstrong seriously in his contention that a certain mathematically-oriented scientism would neglect—or cancel out—the 'visual agency' of the animal gaze and the subjectivity it contains, but we do not need to implicate psychoanalysis, despite its past neglect of the animal, as a field which offers nothing to the study of animal visuality. Lacanian psychoanalytic thought (acting in the same Freudian lineage Armstrong rejects) offers a new approach to this problem that can salvage the animal behind the gaze.

Lacan, in seminar XI, *The Four Fundamental Concepts of Psychoanalysis*, has multiple lectures on the gaze that exceeds—and builds on—his earlier statements on the mirror stage (the specular function) contributing to his overall conception of the imaginary register. In these lectures, Lacan clarifies, in a (seemingly) paradoxical style, that the eye is severed from the gaze—for Lacan, the gaze cannot be reduced to its function as sight, since "I see only from one point, but in my existence I am looked at from all sides."[40] The Lacanian gaze does not follow a unitary outwards-externalized directionality (attached to the eye as that which visualizes) but rather is intractably concomitant with being seen—vision does not delimit the scopic drive, since it includes the various sensory impressions (which Lacan refers to as 'the stain') one leaves on others (those 'actual' individuated others) as well as the Other.[41] This act of being 'seen' or, more precisely gazed upon—subjected to a gaze—is itself not tethered to the visual field: this 'gaze' issues from a locus of presence; the gaze is spatial-sensory awareness of another (Lacan refers to Sartre's conception of the gaze as a 'rustling of leaves,' for instance) or, inversely, being subjected to a gaze is awareness of another's awareness (whether there is a literal manifestation of a gazing 'subject' makes no difference).

Lacan relates this function of the scopic field to castration and lack—the human subject, anchored to their unitary 'gaze' of vision-sight, lacks the perspective of this universalized, multi-directional gaze from which there is no elision (the subject is subjected to a gaze that implacably exceeds their own, "castrating" them from this globalized-microscopic view that the subject furtively "tries to adapt himself to")[42]—and, because these formations are dependent on the symbolic (castration and lack both residing within the symbolic field), they are isolated to humans due to their unique position to the signifier. However, animals are not exempt from the gaze's operation as severed from the literal-visual eye: Lacan actually finds animals to be exemplary of this situation of "the pre-existence to the seen of a given-to-be-seen."[43] He isolates animal mimicry, specifically, as a "distinctive example"[44] of the gaze's presupposed (instinctually presumed) totalizing view.

Mimicry, the capacity for an animal to imitate its environment, is seen as indicative of the fact, according to Lacan, that vision presupposes (even instinctually or biologically) an insistent, assumed "all-seeing"[45] gaze that precedes being seen: One will be seen or viewed (in reality or fantasy), even if they do not see what sees them or from where they are gazed upon. Lacan relies on an extraordinary example of simple, non-behavioral, animal mimicry to illustrate this point: The fact that some animals have *ocelli*, that is, circles representative of eyes, such as peacocks, who may have eye-like black circles adorning their large tails. Why do these simulacrums of eyes exist? (They certainly have no visual-sensory function that would grant the animal a new scopic vantage.) Ocelli exist entirely *for the other's presupposed gaze*. Yes, the peacock can see (through actual eyes), but the peacock also presumes (biologically, since these ocelli are genetically coded and form on their tails, irrespective of any conscious effort by the peacock) that they will be subjected to (an)other's gaze—they 'see' that they will be 'seen' by this gaze. While ocelli mimicry in animals is an exceptional example due to its formal representational relation to eyes and reminder of the seen/see, gazed by/gazed at dyad, any form of animal mimicry has embedded within it the other's gaze. Why does an animal adjust their color to adapt to a given environment that they occupy? Precisely because they anticipate that they will be gazed at without particularized knowledge of the one who gazes.

Animal mimicry, to Lacan, is a momentary reference to move onto human psychoanalytic specificity, but he leaves behind residual (though uninterrogated) insights into the visual-scopic field of animality. How can Lacan's comments on animal mimicry orient our thinking on the functioning of the animal's gaze and exceed the mathematical position it occupies in science and the mysteriously inscrutable position it occupies in culture? It tells us that the animal's gaze, in at least some way, operates according to a dyadic structure of the Lacanian gaze: Their vision presumes a gaze from an unseen other. While Lacan does not dwell on this point, animals do indeed experience, to a different degree, the same basic severance of gaze and eye, sight and being-seen that humans do.

In another lecture, Lacan compares animal mimicry enacted by certain crustaceans (the skeleton shrimp carpella) to the human artistic act of producing a painting-picture, explicating that the crustacean "becomes a picture"[46] through taking on the color of a plant that they "settle" among, namely the invertebrate "quasi-plant animal" Bryozoa. As Lacan directly delineates in his lecture "What is a Picture," "mimicry is no doubt the equivalent of the function which, in man, is exercised in painting."[47] Crucially, Lacan defines any picture as a "trap for the gaze,"[48] later clarifying that the gaze which is trapped in the picture is the artist's own, while the spectator's gaze has a more "complex"[49] relationship to the picture's own externalized gaze:

> [the painter] gives something for the eye to feed on, but he invites the person to whom this picture is presented to lay down his gaze there as one lays down one's weapons . . . . Something is given not so much to the gaze as to the eye.[50]

This "pacifying"[51] function of the painting relates immediately to mimicry: Mimicry offers itself up to the eye (is detected in the visual register) in order to negate the predator gaze; mimicry, like painting, supplants being subjected to the (predatorial) gaze with being seen. Consider the mimicry of the skeleton shrimp (carpella)—Why do they embody the color of the Bryozoa which surrounds them? It is not to go unseen, but rather to be *seen by the eye but not the gaze*—to elude the predatorial gaze that always-already looks at them 'from all sides.'

Strangely, Lacan denies that the procedure of animal mimicry is "bound up with the needs of survival" and instead posits three categories, according to the work of Roger Caillois, through which mimicry functions: "travesty, camouflage, intimidation."[52] As Lacan explicates these 'major dimensions' of mimicry, it becomes apparent they all relate to survival in different degrees of immediacy and efficacy—the commonality which implicitly unites them is their Darwinian-teleological operation that Lacan, seemingly inexplicably, controverts. These three categories—travesty ("disguise, masquerade" for the purpose of "sexual finality"), camouflage ("against a mottled background, of becoming mottled"), and intimidation ("over-valuation that the subject always tries to attain in his appearance"[53] for the other)—all appear in the imaginary.

If we return to Caillois' writings, we see why Lacan rejects the immediate correspondence between mimetic activity and adaptation (for the purpose of survival): Caillois contends in his article "Mimicry and Legendary Psychasthenia" that mimicry has become "the object of those biologists with a heavy predilection for ulterior motives."[54] After enumerating examples of animal mimicry—from caterpillars with eye-like features on their body (the 'inoffensive' animal taking on the appearance of a 'forbidding one') to crabs resembling pebbles (the "adaptation of form to form (homomorphy)" for the purpose of defensive concealment from predators)—Caillois declares the insufficiency of the available biological explanations: "These extreme examples have given rise to numerous attempts at explanation, none of them truly satisfactory."[55]

Caillois contests the conventional biological explanatory mechanism of mimetic activity for survival by first undermining the primacy of sight in predators:

> First of all, it would only apply to carnivores that hunt by sight and not by smell as is often the case. Carnivores, moreover, do not generally bother with motionless prey: immobility would thus be a better defense, and indeed insects are exceedingly prone to employ a false corpselike rigidity.[56]

Later, Caillois finds that the objective facts do not align with the notion of adaption-survival, since "[g]enerally speaking, one finds many remains of mimetic insects in the stomachs of predators" and concludes that mimetic activity, rather than being an instrument of survival, is actually a "dangerous luxury"[57] for the animal. Instead of the adaptation-survival teleological model of mimetic activity, Caillois offers a model predicated on "depersonalization by assimilation to space."[58] He detects in animal mimicry an instinct to collapse "the organism's feeling of distinction from its surroundings"[59]—the animal seeks to assimilate to the background and cease their individuated function as a distinct consciousness in space, instead recoiling into space itself.

Towards the end of his paper, Caillois clarifies that

> it merely suggests that alongside the instinct of self-preservation, which in some way orients the creature toward life, there is generally speaking a sort of instinct of renunciation that orients it toward a mode of reduced existence, which in the end would no longer know either consciousness or feeling.[60]

Mimicry is self-dissolution through embeddedness in what one is not—in what should be other-from-oneself, namely the environment which surrounds them. In short, somewhat astoundingly, Caillois identifies what could be considered a death instinct recognizable in the scopic register: animal mimetic activity is involved, according to Caillois, with an attenuation of existence and consciousness as much as it is self-preservation. Here, we can begin to understand Lacan's claims on painting, animal mimicry, and the gaze—morphological mimicry is not merely to 'lay down' the predatorial gaze embedded into animal instinct, but even to radically reduce the gaze of life itself: to no longer be seen by that which 'sees on all sides'—which exceeds ('little o') 'other' predators—the larger 'Other' that grounds life itself.

If we return to Freud's writing on the death instinct in *Beyond the Pleasure Principle*, we find a similar postulation to Caillois conjecture on mimicry; Freud detects a corresponding tension between self-preservation and self-dissolution across the litany of life throughout the animal kingdom. Freud patently states that the first instinct that came into being, in any living organism, is "the instinct to return to the inanimate state"[61]—he even goes so far as to define instincts (though these should actually be called drives, as he used the word *triebe*) themselves as "*an urge inherent in organic life to restore an earlier state of things*,"[62] and since the original state of animate beings must have been inanimate matter, there is thus an 'inherent' compulsion to 'restore' that original condition which preceded life itself. This compulsion-towards-death can be found in the compulsion to repeat: Freud refers to the migratory practices of birds and fish who, despite the (lack of) evolutionary utility of doing so, return to a similar place—he finds that this compulsion to repeat is a basic instinct to 'return' that is 'conservative' rather than 'progressive' (progressive and conservative here referring to expending libidinal economy either towards evolutionary self-preservation or in the opposite direction, towards self-dissolution); the compulsion to repeat does not seek to move life into a new adaptive space, but instead to return to an older space—a position, if sufficiently reached, towards death. In a passage that functions as a proper precursor to later implications of the human death drive, Freud writes that "the instinctual life as a whole serves to bring about death";[63] however, because every organism "wishes to die only in its own fashion"[64] there remains a lingering counter libidinal-economic investment in self-preservation that impedes the instinctual restoration of the original inanimate state: there are "life instincts and death instincts"[65] working in immediately oppositional directions—eros and thanos.

At this juncture, the relation between Lacan, Caillois, and the Freudian 'death drive' should be clear: Lacan observes, in the visual-scopic field (according to Caillois' conception of mimetic activity as an 'assimilation' to space and mimetic animals thus becoming a site of indistinction with their spatial environment in an attempt to attenuate consciousness) a purposive elision of the gaze that has no adaptive-survival function for the individual nor the species. Lacan's remarks on animality and the gaze situate a death instinct within the animal-imaginary register: There is an impulse, though, as I will explicate in later chapters, not quite an instinct, according to Lacan (informed by Caillois' insights) that causes animal's to utilize the visual field (of potentially presupposed Other who looks 'from all sides') in the diminution of their own existence—and, definitionally, these 'instincts' can be assigned the Freudian name of a death drive issuing from the Other.

Lacan's thoughts on animal mimicry and the non-adaptive procedure of the gaze present a radical break with current biological and ethological models of understanding animal mimicry. Contemporary animal researchers, operating according to the "predilection" for "ulterior motives" that Caillois consigns them, have further solidified the relationship between evolutionary adaptation and mimicry. The consensus among scientists is that mimicry "must be adaptive."[66] However, at the margins of mimetic activity across animals, we find behaviors that seem to negate precisely that pre-assumed scientific consensus. Biologists have detected seemingly non-adaptive activities like “imperfect mimics,” where an animal’s mimetic output “resemble their models imprecisely,”[67] resulting in a mimetic effect that is ineffectual (in terms of corresponding to the model-material the animal mimics) yet is concurrently consistent across the species (meaning it is not a mere individual physio-genetic aberration). In these cases, such as non-venomous snakes who hold a “coarse resemblance” to “highly venomous coral snakes,”[68] the mimetic activity does not sufficiently act to result in an adaptive advantage and augment the chances of survival for either the species or the individual animal.

While many researchers attempt to reconcile these non-adaptive mimetic activities and the tenets of purely progressive evolutionism, claiming, for instance, that imperfect mimics are caused by developmental constraints which stunt the ability to “evolve a closer match to the model,” which is, likely, eventually “overcome”[69] after a given duration of time. Objections exist, such as we have seen by Lacan and Caillois, that demand a reappraisal of the adaptive functioning of mimesis.

Lacan’s visual-scopic remarks on animality and the procedure of the gaze in no way undermine evolution as a theory of animal development—it simply complicates the notions of animal consciousness, instincts, and the visual field. Animal instincts and physio-genetic development are not taken, in Lacan’s view, to exist in a unilinear unfolding across temporality; instead, animals are found to participate in an ambivalent, non-progressive relation to life-and-death which is normally only ascribed to the human (although this view, somewhat prophetically, is found in the originary texts on the death drive from Freud himself).

The Other of Animality: The Imaginary Other and the PredaOther

Lacan, at one point, demarcates between the insights of the specular mirror-image function and the ‘all-seeing’ gaze he establishes in *The Four Fundamental Concepts of Psychoanalysis*. As noted in the preceding section, the specular self-reflexive image’s procedure coheres the multiplicity of the body into a unified totality (however, this totality is alienating, and as Lacan writes in his critique of the cogito, it is even self-delusory). Because the mirror-stage is predicated on the externalized-outer line of sight, in which “as soon as I perceive, my representations belong to me,”[70] there is an adoption of the mirror-image (an identification). For the gaze, we see the exact opposite: There is not an adoption (an identification, a form of ownership); there is, rather, an *adaptation* (conforming to the gaze’s demand). The impact of this notion of gaze on a field such as film studies is clear—the gaze is taken to be determinative for the one-who-is-gazed-upon (the actress, for instance); the one who is subject to the gaze comports to that gaze (and from there a popular branch of feminist film criticism emerges, facilitated by Laura Mulvey’s famous essay). Consider adaptation in the dimension that Lacan denies (the most immediate, scientific-evolutionary sense): A given animal who-is-gazed-upon by the predator comports to the predatorial gaze by deploying mimesis to elude that very gaze—the crucial insight here is that despite the attempt to avoid this gaze, the gaze is nonetheless determinative of the mimetic behavior on a physio-genetic level.

But what does this tell us about the content of the animal gaze itself—of the gaze that issues from an animal, rather than merely the inescapable gaze an animal anticipates being subjected to? We should not expect to perfectly fill in the individuated subjectivity transmitted by an animal—yet, like Lacan's psychoanalytic treatment of humans, we can outline the structural arrangement which governs the gaze of animals and the scopic field's network, thereby stretching the knowledge of animal subjectivity in new, un-explored, territorialities. Broadly, we can classify animals into three Lacanian imaginary taxonomies: Those animals who participate in the specular function and are subjected to the all-seeing gaze (*specular animals subject to gaze*); those animals who do not participate in the specular function and *are* subjected to the all-seeing gaze (*non-specular animals subject to gaze*); and, finally, those animals who neither participate in the specular function nor are subjected to the all-seeing gaze (*non-specular animals not subject to gaze*). Largely, these categories correspond to already-established biological-cognitive categories—those animals capable of bodily self-consciousness and higher degrees of self-awareness (apes, monkeys, dolphins, etc.) would align with *specular animals subject to gaze*, while pigeons, who are incapable of the specular function (do not relate a pre-lingual self to the self-same image in the mirror) but are subject to the gaze (which is evident through their engagement in mimicry) could be codified as *non-specular animals subject to gaze*, and those animal-beings who neither recognize their body in the mirror nor exhibit awareness of a gaze, such as the 'quasi-animal' Bryozoa which Lacan references, would correspond to the category of *non-specular animals not subject to gaze*.

The imaginary taxonomies (extrapolated from Lacan's own comments on the visual function in animals) define the visual dyad of seeing/being seen and supply insights into subjective investments in the scopic field: Knowing that an animal recognizes the gaze of another (or potentially an-Other), themselves-as-themselves (the specular function of bodily-self recognition), or neither, certainly furnishes an entry-point to a psychoanalytic interiority of animality. We begin to see that, while psychoanalytic activity occurs in the linguistic register in the case of the human, for animals, psychoanalytic activity conversely transpires in the visual (or, in a larger sense, imaginary-sensory) field. While we must refrain from establishing a fixed, stable hierarchy of animality and their respective attributes, the contours of these classifications (which surely could be contested if mis-taken as eternal demarcations or biological categories) lead to a deeper psychoanalytic-philosophical understanding of the visual field of animality and a corresponding subjectivity.

To illustrate the non-fixed nature of these Lacanian taxonomies: It remains entirely open, for instance, whether a *specular animal not subject to gaze* is a categoric possibility. Could there be an animal who participates in the specular function yet is somehow not subject to the gaze? This seems, from the outset, an undeniably resolute impossibility—it would appear that the cognitive capacity for bodily self-consciousness would preclude one from inaccessibility to the gaze. If one recognizes themselves, they must recognize that they are seen by others; if an animal who does not recognize itself can recognize *being seen*, then the ability for visual self-recognition in the scopic field must bring with it, in an implicit, automatic, and latent manner, the ability to know that one is seen. Yet, there remains, unexamined and thereby unexhausted, the prospect of an animal that can do just that—or an animal whose being is precisely that.

If animals are subject to the gaze, and the gaze issues, according to Lacan, from the "field of the Other,"[71] then must animals have an Other which submits them to the gaze? Clearly, there is something analogous in animals to the human ('big O') Other. However, as established in Chapter 1, there is not the symbolic framework in place for animals that is needed to constitute a place for the Other to occupy. As Lacan insists, the Other exists in the symbolic register—to be precise, the Other is the grounding for the symbolic domain; the human Other is concurrently predicated on and constituted by an interplay (a transsubjective exchange) of signifiers and is the regulatory nexus of the signifier (its Law). For Lacan, the (human) Other is "defined as the site of speech"[72]—it is not "where speech is uttered, but where it takes on the value of speech."[73] The Other is not synonymous with the place where language emanates from in the act of speech—the human subject (the site of enunciation "where speech is uttered")—conversely, the Other is the transsubjective "site" where speech "takes on the value of speech." All speech is "verified" in the "locus"[74] of the Other. This site is, notably, foreign to the subject: It is language, not in terms of a static or even ever-expanding and contracting 'objective' lexicon which acts as a collective repository of words and their usage-status, but the novel, entirely individuated language one encounters as they subjectively pass through the world. A human being is dropped into this Other, already developed and totally severed from them, and then, as one encounters this already-existing Other of language, it accrues in the subject through a ceaseless series of encounters—here we see that the Other occupies the strange, paradoxical status as absolutely foreign and alienating, as well as intimately embedded in oneself (and, not to delude the reader, even as this alienating Other is embedded deeply into the human subject, it maintains its position of alterity—becoming the very site we know as the 'unconscious').

When Lacan writes that the gaze 'issues' from the Other, one should understand this as the human Other, which is an inter-bounded confluence of the symbolic and imaginary domains (the register of the Real is also present, but I will suspend its introduction until the next chapter)—for the human, the imaginary cannot be severed from the symbolic: the visual field, once one irrevocably enters the symbolic via the signifier (once the subject speaks), is experienced through the prism of the symbolic register. As Jacques-Alain Miller writes in *Paradigms of Jouissance*, "the imaginary is clearly that which remains outside the grasp of the symbolic," yet "Lacan always writes that this imaginary is at the same time dominated by the symbolic."[75] When one begins to speak, what one sees and identifies with (in the register of the imaginary) is seen in the tint of language: the visual scene is transmuted by the signifier. There are, of course, already illusory elements constitutively embedded in vision which structure our experience of the visual dimension (our spatial-visual reality), and the symbolic acts as the immanent terrain for processing the visual. Pure, direct access to a given visual object—for the human—is always a fiction due to the interference from the scopic function itself and the symbolic.

While this is the condition for humans and their Other, different conditions are at play for animals, who are alienated from the symbolic register. For them, there appears to be an Other independent of the signifier—we find, in animals (those who are subject to the gaze), that there is an *imaginary Other* which haunts their visual-subjective field. In Seminar V, *Formation of the Unconscious*, while discussing Pavlovian behavioral experiments, Lacan provides a useful hint towards a conception of the animal Other:

> no matter how far these experiments are taken, what is not found, and perhaps what there is no question of finding, is the law under which these signifiers which are brought into play, are ordered, and which amounts to saying that it is the law which in the long run animals obey. It is quite clear in fact that there is no trace of a reference to such a law, namely to anything which is beyond a signal, or that from a short chain of signals once established, no sort of legalizing extrapolation, is perceptible in it, and this is indeed why one can say that one never succeeds in establishing the law. I repeat: this is not to say for all that that there is no dimension of the Other with a capital O for the animal. Nothing is effectively articulated within qua discourse.[76]

At the start, there is a sentiment present similar to what Lacan subsequently rearticulated in Seminar XX: the signifier—which is a signifier for the human—is a sign for an animal; the animal interacts with the signifier (through the behavioral experiment, mediated by the researchers), but there is no animal-internal 'law' to order it structurally, and accordingly the signifier falls into its function as a 'signal' for the animal. The end of the quote, though it is not a path that Lacan fully pursues (as we've seen with his commentary on animals, he uses them either as a fleeting referential site or as a illustrative digressions towards his insights on human psychoanalytic matters), does puncture the discourse on animals: While one might assume that Lacan's attestation of animals' non-access to the symbolic would render them, in turn, "Other-less," Lacan conversely gestures towards an opening for an animal Other. He plainly refuses to deny animals a "dimension of the Other with a capital O."[77]

How should one take Lacan's enigmatic statement on the animal and the Other? It is clear, for the animal, that the Other is not tethered to the symbolic as it is for the human being (as the beginning of the quote outlines)—yet this leaves us with no register in which to situate the animal's Other, and there would thus be no way to form a Lacanian conception of this animal dimension. However, when one returns to a quote cited at the start of the chapter, from *The Four Fundamental Concepts of*

Psychoanalysis, we are reminded that animals are (largely) "caught up" in an "imaginary capture"[78]—we must note that the status of animals being fully "caught up" is certainly contestable, as I posited in the preceding chapter through animal access to the sign (and thus qualify through the parenthetical 'largely') but nonetheless, here we detect a Lacanian register to situate the animal Other: For the animal, it is an *imaginary Other*—or, put more simply, it is an Other in the imaginary (rather than symbolic) register. Here, we find ourselves at (what appears to be) an immoderate departure from Lacan's writings—he never ventured to locate an Other outside of the symbolic which, according to his thought, would be strictly impossible, but it must be recognized that a non-symbolic Other is only an impossibility *for the human*, the being who employs the signifier's arbitrary vessel as opposed to a sign.

The animal's imaginary Other, like the human symbolic Other, is a structural nexus site of organizational Law: If the human Other is the 'site of speech,' then the animal Other is the 'site of the image.' One should observe here that the human Other is not the site of the signifier (the constitutive component of speech), and, similarly, the animal Other is not the site of the optical-scopic process (the apparatus that permits the emergence of image)—both Others exist at *the point in which an individuated subjectivity encounters the world*. At these junctures, the encounter with the world (whether that world is perceived in its symbolic or imaginary dimensions) forms an alterity that is privatized in the subject. Due to the fact that human experience is structured by the symbolic, we have privileged language and either attempted to accentuate language-ability in animals (the deluge of texts claiming to map animal language—really only delineating communicative mechanisms, functioning according to codes or signs, utterly distinct from what we mean by 'language') or assumed that animal experience is non-mediated (in the non-biological, psychoanalytic sense) by any dimension and is immersed in an uninterpretable immediacy.

Consider the notion of a language-less being in a phenomenological sense: What would it mean to exist without language? For the human, access to some postulated, pure languageless dimension is definitionally inconceivable in Lacanian thought (although it is true that the Real acts as an 'impossible' puncture of the symbolic)—and because of this, we perceive a subjectivity not submitted through the symbolic (a conscious existent independent of language) as unmediated by anything: Without language, we assume that experience itself must be known in all its immediacy; encounters with the world must be—because they are not submitted to the prism of language—left unchanged aside from the perceptual-sensory processes natural distortions (olfactory, tactile, auditory, gustatory, and visual systems and their inexorable alterations to 'raw' reality). This presupposition is precisely the error theorists insist on when approaching animality. The assertion that animals have direct access to something which eludes humans; *therefore*, it is assumed that their experience is totally unstructured aside from some bio-genetic instinctiveness. Animals are not, however, unanchored by anything, nor are they totally captured by instincts; their experience is mediated by the imaginary register—by the scopic-visual field which structures their subjectivity. For animals, the image is Law. Importantly, as Lacan clarifies, the imaginary does not permit a direct immediacy—there is a lack in the image: "image is characterized by a lack, that is, by the fact that what is called upon there is unable to appear there."[79] There is an untraversable split between the world of the imaginary and the world of objective reality—the imaginary mediates, and introduces a lack (though, as I explicate later, this lack is distinct from human lack—it may be preferable, and more accurate, to refer to animal lack as a condition of non-totality or non-immediacy), into animal subjectivity.

Conceiving of subjectivity—of animal interiority—as structured by the image is not some radical theoretical claim unsubstantiated by positivist science: It corresponds perfectly to contemporary research attempting to penetrate the very meaning of animal consciousness itself. Animal neurobiologist Michael Land explicitly links the visual field to consciousness, writing that "consciousness arises in brain structures that analyse the attributes of the external world, such as colour, depth, and motion, then it seems reasonable to think that whatever analyses of similar complexity are carried out they too will be accompanied by conscious awareness."[80] For humans, language mediates this analysis of the external world's attributes—as Lacan says, "[i]t is the world of words that creates the world of things"[81]—the symbolic Other "creates" the "world of things" that humans come to inhabit. In this case, conscious awareness (the process of perceiving and analyzing the empirical, objective world) is refracted through the symbolic register. For animals, there is still a mediation of "the world of things"—in the imaginary rather than symbolic register: in animal subjectivity *it is the world of images that creates the world of things*. The attributes of the external world are refracted through the Law of the image.

The scopic function—and the operation of the imaginary Other—in animals is a site of subjectivity rather than a site of instinctiveness (which would, crucially, be devoid of any 'subject'). Simply, the visual field dominates, and even 'structures,' the animal experience, but this does not denote a centralized, autonomous subject. Again, Land provides an apt insight into the visual function in animals that contend, in an indirect manner, with this objection: "With the evolution of complex vision has come the need to choose between different behaviors. Such choices need to be managed by an 'oversight' system, and that would seem to involve conscious visual experience."[82] Land claims that the existence of a 'complex' visual system, embedded in an animal's bio-physical organization and modifying their phenomenological access to empirical reality, causes a proliferation of choices (based on the various things to be seen) which necessitate a consciousness to select among the available acts. Instincts do, doubtlessly, inform the impulse to flee when an animal is confronted with a danger (as they do for humans), but there must be some oversight apparatus which selects *among the variety of choices* as those choices become more complex. If an animal concurrently sees an attractive mate and a predator, they do not proceed to *flee and mate* at the same time (albeit these two instincts would certainly be present); there is an overseeing apparatus (which we can call consciousness, or more contentiously, subjectivity) that analyzes the visual data and accordingly *acts*.

The relation of the animal to gaze and the specular field functions as a cleavage, a theoretical entry-site, into the animal (imaginary) Other. Lacan's pigeons, for instance, are exemplary of the Law of image and the imaginary Other. Recall that the female pigeon enters maturation through the assimilation-of-the-other's image. This intervention, enacted through the sight of another, is structured around an image. However, while this zoological insight from Lacan is frequently cited, it is ordinarily only contended with as an analog for understanding Lacan's concept of the mirror stage in human development, as formulated in his essay "The Mirror Stage as Formative of the I Function."

Lacan derives his views on female pigeons and visuality from Leonard Harrison Matthews' short (only four-page) paper, "Visual Stimulation and Ovulation in Pigeon," published in 1938. In his paper, Matthews provides a brief overview of experiments involving pigeons and corresponding insights on sexual maturation. He begins the article with an insistent line, appearing to relay a consensus: "It has long been known that the female pigeon, unlike the carefully selected domestic hen, does not ovulate spontaneously."[83] Instead of female pigeons ovulating "spontaneously," he asserts, according to an experiment that placed pigeons in cages, some paired and others isolated, that "results obtained show that the stimulus which causes ovulation in the pigeon is a visual one" and that "visual stimulation from a companion of the same sex, or even from a mirror image visual stimulation from a companion of the same sex, or even from a mirror image, is sufficient to produce ovulation."[84]

A rodent that primarily resides in Europe, the female bank vole, also exhibits the function of the image in sexual reproduction, but in the opposing direction: Research has shown that "pregnancy in female bank voles can be blocked if the females are exposed early in the pregnancy to the pheromones from a male bank vole that is not the father."[85] In this instance, quite comparable to pigeon gonad development, there is an olfactory 'image' at play that is determinative of pregnancy—the image-of-another-who-is-not-the-father prevents the production of offspring. The scent-image, on the plane of the olfactory system using the coordinates of pheromones, directs the proliferation of animal *life itself.* What is truly confounding about the bank vole is that the imaginary radically contravenes the instinctual evolutionary force of reproduction—the image overcomes the putative orientation of all animal behavior and bodily functions towards the end of self-conservation and self-perpetuation through offspring. Even if there is an evolutionarily advantageous reason covertly hidden behind the operation of the image, it is entirely auxiliary to the insight that animal subjectivity and behavior is structured by the imaginary field and its network of identifications (it is through the imaginary that the female bank vole recognizes the father and the not-father).

In his seminal work *Attachment*, John Bowlby tells us how attachment between animals—such as that between mother and infant—is developed according to "specificity":

> Often within hours of hatching eggs or giving birth to young, a parent can distinguish its own young from any others and then will behave parentally only to

> them; the young in their turn come to distinguish their own parents a from all other adults and thenceforward behave in a special way towards them.[86]

What field can possibly permit this recognition of specificity? It is precisely the imaginary register—that of the image-of-another—which brings parent and child into proximity. An example Bowlby relies on is the "vocal call"[87] of the young, attracting the parent to them—and this certainly operates in the imaginary field (it is a sonic image of the child). Bowlby finds that "individual recognition and highly differentiated behavior are, then, the rule in the parent-young relations of birds and mammals."[88] Not much, if anything, has changed this "rule" in the intervening years since Bowlby's study of attachment behaviors.

Similarly, defensive-protective mimicry in animals, deployed to coalesce with one's background, for instance—operating for a non-specific (predatorial) gaze—is evidence of the imaginary Other. What is this presupposed predatorial gaze (that notably does not issue from an individuated animal but rather from an *anticipated* predator irreducible to any one animal—or even to any numerical set of animals; a gaze 'from all sides' without correspondence to eyes) if not the interiority of an animal's imaginary displaced into the world? Predator(s) certainly objectively exist and undeniably threaten the prey animal's actual existence—yet it should be equally transparent that the anticipated predatorial gaze exists within the interiority of the animal, in their very subjectivity, spurring their mimetic activity. At this point, there is utility in distinguishing between a predator and the *predaOther*: The predator sees through localized eyes with all their inherent constraints of scope; the predaOther 'sees' in absence of eyes and is scopeless, limitless, and inescapable. The animal can elude the predator's line of localized sight but cannot elude the predaOther's gaze.

For an animal subjected to gaze, whether or not they participate in the specular function, the predaOther has an immanent structural procedure in subjectivity. When Lacan describes the human subject's relation to the "scopic drive," he writes that humans are "beings who are looked at, in the spectacle of the world"[89] and "[f]rom the moment this gaze appears, the subject tries to adapt himself to it, he becomes the punctiform object."[90] This is why, as Lacan explains, certain animals, such as the skeleton shrimp "carpella" he relies on as an example, "becomes a picture"[91] through their mimetic activity—not because they are gazed upon by the same Other as humans (the symbolic Other), but because they are gazed upon by this expansive and inexhaustible predaOther. One must recall, of course, that the gaze is never (for the human or the animal) centralized in a "subject to subject"[92] relation, since that visual exchange would occur on the horizon of the eye, rather than the gaze, and would remain affixed to "the existence of others looking at me."[93] This is precisely why the gaze "appears to us as all-seeing"[94]—because it is a gaze of interiority externalized, only occasionally aligning, or appearing to align (as a fantasy), with the actual sight of others. The gaze—issued from the (symbolic) Other—"intervenes"[95] in the human subject "in a function of desire" in order for the subject to sustain themselves: The Other's gaze structures the subject's desire (and desire is, for the human, the founding of the subject-as-subject, causing him to act). For animals, the Other's gaze serves a similar function.

The predaOther formally illustrates, as does the female pigeon's gonad maturation instigated by visual stimulation, the structural effects of the imaginary: In both instances, the animal's being conforms to a certain subjective ratification of (imaginary) Law determined by the visual field. The visual, for many animals, is not merely a sensory organ—it is, rather, the primary mode through which their subjectivity is issued through; animal subjectivity is constituted by the imaginary field. The exact questions one would pose to humans and their relation to language (the Lacanian symbolic) can be posed to animals and their relation to the visual-scopic function: How is 'raw' reality altered through this function? Is the notion of an animal subjectivity conceivable—in the same sense—in absence of this function? The imaginary entails a series of identifications and associations—and animal consciousnesses are determined by these series. For a specular animal subject to gaze, such as a dolphin, ape, or monkey, they participate in the non-lingual visual self-identification as well as the species-level identification (to capitulate to language: 'that is me' and 'that is one of my kind'). Identification, engendered through the imaginary, is the defining structural framework of any animal consciousness: An animal subjectivity is imaginary, whether they have bodily self-consciousness (specular animal subjected to gaze) or are a non-specular animal subjected to gaze (meaning they *adapt* to the imaginary association of the predaOther).

One could object here: What about the animal who does not rely on the visual dimension? Do they not negate this very notion of the imaginary Other and the predaOther? One should be reminded that the gaze is irreducible to the function of the eye, as Lacan clearly posits: "must we not distinguish between the function of the eye and that of the gaze?"[96] On one level, as has already been observed, this demarcation is necessary to distinguish between the sight of others (issuing from eyes) and the gaze of the Other (issuing from no-eyes). Both the animal Other and human Other are not merely visual transmissions from the optical sites of (lower 'o') other subjects. Further, the imaginary is not totally bound by the visual function; the gaze entirely exceeds visuality. When discussing the gaze in Sartre's work, Lacan deftly observes,

> If you turn to Sartre's own text, you will see that, far from speaking of the emergence of this gaze as something that concerns the organ of sight, he refers to the sounds of rustling leaves, suddenly heard while out hunting, to a footstep heard in a corridor.[97]

The gaze is not limited to visuality—and the animal who lacks visuality (or the animal in which visuality is not situated in a position of absolute primacy), does not lack a sense of the gaze. Unlike a predator, the predaOther looks but is never seen (and thus does not rely on sight). Non-visual emergences, such as 'the rustling of leaves' or a 'footstep,' occurring in the sonic domain, are reminders that signify the predaOther's all-seeing imaginary gaze. The imaginary Other surpasses simple relegation to the scopic drive—a sightless animal still experiences this phenomenon of being seen from a non-specific vantage, and this is precisely how mimetic sonic activity emerges, such as the Lyrebird's ability to reflect a range of noises to dissuade predators mimetically. Sound acts as a signal of the gaze (as Lacan illustrates with the rustling leaves), and sound is conversely an instrument of dispelling, of breaking the gaze of the imaginary Other: What is the implicit operation in the sonic mimetic activity of a Lyrebird if not conforming (adapting) to a predaOther's gaze (which, notably, preexists any individual predator)?

We have discovered, then, two stratums of the Other: The symbolic Other (the Other of humanity) and the imaginary Other (the Other of animality). Both Others adhere to a binding operation in the respective subjects, with the subject adapting themself to the gaze which issues from the "field of the Other."[98] To arrive at the true insight, it must be observed that this ability to detect the contour of animal experience—to pinpoint the imaginary Other, the predaOther, and classify animals' specular and non-specular functions—is immeasurably distinct from the presupposition that animals present a site of absolute opacity, an inexplicable and inscrutable density of consciousness (or pre-consciousness), without an emission permitting any human-epistemic access. Rather, we see that animals *can* be approached as subjects and that the contents of their experience can be submitted to psychoanalytic, particularly Lacanian, knowledge. Animals contain an interiority—a subjectivity—and this subjectivity can be known in its structural imaginary dimension: an animal can be known as a psychoanalytic subject beyond the law of the signifier.

Love in the Imaginary: Animal Love Without a Signifier

In the preceding chapter on the symbolic, I ended by commenting on Lacan's seemingly cryptic note at the conclusion of Seminar XX on the limits of knowledge, the symbolic, recognition of presence, and the corresponding implications for animal love. There, I found that the dog's bark functions as a sign of love via declaration of intersubjective self-presence alongside the relationship between the sign and guilt—and, of course, as Freud reminds us, the psychoanalytic fact that love is always implicated in guilt. It is lucidly transparent, as I observed in the first chapter, that love as such does not solely inhabit the symbolic field—it, instead, eludes the symbolic by residing in those registers which exceed or are inaccessible to it: the registers of the Real and the imaginary. To seize this thread which was begun in the foregoing chapter: If (some) animals can be conferred the capacity of love—an embedded *desire*—then how does this love-ability relate to the imaginary function for animals, such as the imaginary Other and the predaOther?

In Bruce Fink's book *Lacan on Love*, he discusses love in the imaginary register by beginning with the "importance of images for triggering significant developmental processes"[99] in animals. Fink asserts, as we have established, that the imaginary field holds a crucial position in the experience of animals. Later, he addresses the "importance of images in courting and mating behavior in the animal kingdom."[100] Upon arriving at the mirror stage, Fink sharply distinguishes between the animal and the human since humans only "function as a unit" through a mirrored image of themselves that "gives or reflects back to the child an image of its own body as whole"[101]—while the animal undergoes a development that "occurs automatically over the course of time."[102] As mentioned earlier, humans experience a psychic totality (the threshold of the ego-self) through the self-assumed mirror-image that offers an "artificial unity"[103] preceding an actual functional unity. To make this point, Fink relies on Lacan's ethological assumptions, according to the research available to him, that animals such as chimpanzees were unable to recognize themselves in a mirror. Conversely, as established earlier in this chapter, studies have found that monkeys can be trained to recognize themselves in the mirror and do, indeed, have bodily self-consciousness. While Fink supplies perceptive insights into Lacan's work and explicates Lacanian ideas, his fidelity to Lacanian thought (to explaining what Lacan *meant*) results in eliding over the fact that Lacan's writings are, occasionally, circumscribed by the time they were written—especially when involving non-psychoanalytic or philosophical fields such as ethology and zoology which were still settling their proper scientific foundations. (It must be noted, though, that at the time Fink's book was published, the study on monkey self-recognition I cite had not yet become available.)

Accordingly, as Fink continues in his chapter on the imaginary and Lacanian love, he leaves behind animality in a pre-specular domain—he notes that the image is significant to their development, yet indicates they have no place in proper imaginary identification:

> The process of human 'development'—unlike what we see in animal development—thus jumps from inadequacy (the-body-in-pieces, the body as fragmented, ununified, and an "original disarray" or jumble . . .) to anticipated wholeness: an artificial or anticipated unity prior to real unity (somewhat akin to the reunification of Germany—an artificial unity is created at a national level long before any kind of real social, cultural, or economic unity has been achieved).[104]

Fink explains that there is no need for this artificial unity in animality since there is already a functional unity; the development of animal's act as an inversion of his Germany reunification analogy: A country with real functional unity ("social, cultural, or economic unity") has no need of an artificial psychic unity (the 'national' unity). While the elided constitutive developmental phase (or 'stage' in Lacan's lexicon) of artificial, subjective unity through self-recognition in an imaginary image has certain implications for the formation of an animal ego, we cannot neglect the variance across animality of bodily self-consciousness, and consequently, subjective unity. Here, one must instead include (some) animals in a specular imaginary-identificatory function. Simply, there are some animals who engage in the specular function and, despite not having the same developmental position that the 'mirror stage' has for humans and the construction of their ego, self-recognition within the mirror indicates a participation in the very imaginary self-identification that Fink (following Lacan) restricts to humans.

In terms of love-ability (as in the ability to give, rather than be the recipient of, love), this leaves a few empty spaces where certain animals can enter: After leaving animals behind in pre-specularity, Fink discusses the ideal-ego as

> the external point or place from which [the child] is seen as lovable by the parent, and thereby comes to see itself as if it were itself in the parent's position . . . the point at which one is viewed as worthwhile by the Other.[105]

Regardless of the fact that the gesture which spurs this ideal-ego (the parent's 'nod' or other act of recognition as the baby sees themself in a mirror—a 'ratification' of the mirror image) has a unique specificity in the development of the human, there remains a slit from which the animal can be seen to participate in this same self-identification with the 'point' (the site of the Other) by which they are 'seen as lovable.'

To again reference the dog's guilt from Chapter 1: When the dog chews on the shoe, and no one is home (and we can certainly infer that the dog indeed has knowledge of a human abstention), from what vantage is their guilt imposed? Do we assume that this guilt only appears in the presence of the human via their arrival into the home? No, the dog's guilt, following the act, precedes the human's arrival into the home—*since it is issued from the Other* (this Other being, again, irreducible to any given person's presence—albeit an individuated other can certainly be representative of this Other, as the parents are for the child or the owner is for the dog) and, similar to the procedure it holds in the ego-ideal in the child in relation to their (m)Other, this Other is a locus of lovability (the source of love, issues exogenously from an external site). Fink explains, following Lacan, that "the Other's approving gaze at oneself is brought inside, as it were, and one begins to view oneself approvingly as the Other views one (the Other's disapproving gaze will, of course, come into play as well)."[106] Lacan explicitly links the operation of the Other to the dog's relation to their owner during his seminar on Anxiety, stating that, "When you know how a dog behaves vis-a-vis the one who calls himself, or doesn't, his master, you know that in every case the dimension of the Other counts for a dog."[107] There is an installed sense of the image of oneself as seen by the Other for the dog in relation to his or her "master." When the owner's gaze (functioning in the imaginary domain) along with complementary signifiers—such as 'bad dog!' (a signifier which for the dog is received as a sign, primarily subsisting in the imaginary)—is broadcast towards the dog, they take on this image that is reflected in their guilt when the disapproved act is repeated.

Although I am not, necessarily, claiming that the dog is participating in the exact same complex self-identification procedure of the ego-ideal (since this may involve a deeper self-understanding and established egoic system that potentially exceeds the dog's sense of self and Other)—I am positing that the dog's guilt situates their being in an interplay of the (animal) self and the Other which constitutes a network of love. Wynne and Udel even attempt to reclassify what is ostensibly 'guilt' in a dog as 'appeasement' or 'fearful behavior':

> In other words, your dog may not be so guilty after all—instead it may just be responding to your scolding behaviors—the tone of your voice, the way your hands are placed on your tops just so, or the tap of your foot.[108]

Although we should be critical of the attempt to reclassify the dog's behavior as not constituting guilt, since externally-imposed fear is precisely where Freud argues guilt emerges from (it seems that Wynee and Udel do not distinguish between what I would refer to as externalized first-order guilt and superegoic second-order guilt), what are these gestures the dog fears if not the gaze of the Other instantiated by the owner? In the triangulation of the dog and the owner, there is a third party—the Other in the purely imaginary register—through which the dog views themselves as lovable or unlovable, loved or unloved. The ideal-self (or, if we can perhaps hesitantly refer to this as a diluted animal ideal-ego) of the 'good dog' (albeit the phonological elements themselves are certainly meaningless for the dog) is punctured through the gaze cast from the actual locus of the Other (the owner). Lacan seems to indicate exactly this, delineating the function of the "good object" as an "image" that "makes the dog faithful."[109] The dog is faithful in order to take on the image of the "good object" for the Other—and the image of the "good object" is reflected back to the dog by the owner's own image. As we see in Fink's elaboration on the imaginary and ego-identification there is an "*internationalization* . . . there being henceforward an ideal image or set of images that structures one's sense of self."[110] For the dog, this is not bound to the mirrored self-image, but rather the imaginary Other—in this case, the image of the Other via the owner's smile or grimace, softness of tone or depth of shout, verbal transmission of 'good dog' or 'bad dog' (received by the dog as signs in the imaginary). This Other's image "structures one's sense of self" regardless of the absence, for the dog, of a literal specular image of oneself.

Visuality is tied to the dog's self through the Other—and this further uncovers the animal relation to love: the dog (like other animals) experiences, and directly expresses, guilt engendered by the loss of the ideal-image of themselves that the reception of the Other's image brings. If love could be, very roughly, and admittedly incompletely, defined as attachment which exceeds bio-need, we find here a perfect instance of love in animality: The loss for the dog is not the food which the owner brings, but rather the *image of oneself as lovable by the Other*. For, if one would object that the owner is connected to bio-need due to being the source of food—consider the position of the parent of a human: Are they not, also, the source of sustenance for the child? Yet, for the human child, we see that the loss (of the ego-ideal) exceeds the loss of sustenance; it is the loss of the very image of oneself as lovable by the Other. Here we locate the opposing functions of the owner-Other and the predaOther: the predaOther is the image which structures the fear-response and the owner-Other is that which structures the love-response.

It is, undeniably, advantageous at this point to observe that dogs may represent a special case—possibly through their domesticated relation to humanity—that positions them as an outlier in animality that experiences love. However, in the imaginary taxonomies established, there are animals topographically *more involved* than dogs in terms of their ability to engage in the specular function: If dogs can love, then space is theoretically available for other animals to be ceded the ostensibly human-only territory of love (I leave it up to future multi-disciplinary psychoanalytic zoologists to pursue this line of inquiry further). As for our purposes, animal love has still not been exhausted in Lacanian thought.

Notes

1 Jacques Lacan, *Écrits*, trans. Bruce Fink (New York: W. W. Norton & Company, 2006), 205.
2 Lacan, *Écrits*, 388.
3 Camille Paglia, *Sexual Personae: Art and Decadence from Nefertiti to Emily Dickinson* (New Haven: Yale University Press, 1990), 61.
4 Jacques Lacan, *The Four Fundamental Concepts of Psycho-Analysis: The Seminar of Jacques Lacan, Book XI*, ed. Jacques-Alain Miller, trans. Alan Sheridan (New York: W. W. Norton & Company, 1981), 107.
5 Jacques Derrida, *The Animal That Therefore I Am*, ed. Marie-Louise Mallet, trans. David Wills (New York: Fordham University Press, 2008), 122.
6 Lacan, *Écrits*, 75.
7 Hub Zwart, "Conditioned Reflexes and the Symbolic Order: A Lacanian Assessment of Ivan Pavlov's Experimental Practice," *Vestigia: The Journal of the International Network of Psychotherapeutic Practice* (2018): 4.
8 Liangtang Chang, Shikun Zhang, Mu-ming Poo, and Neng Gong, "Spontaneous Expression of Mirror Self-Recognition in Monkeys after Learning Precise Visual-Proprioceptive Association for Mirror Images," *Proceedings of the National Academy of Sciences* 114, no. 12 (2017): 3258.
9 Chang et al., "Spontaneous Expression of Mirror Self-Recognition," 3262.
10 Chang et al., "Spontaneous Expression of Mirror Self-Recognition," 3258.
11 Lacan, *Écrits*, 77.
12 Lacan, *Écrits*, 77.
13 Peter Buse, "The Dog and the Parakeet: Lacan Among the Animals," *Angelaki: Journal of Theoretical Humanities* 22, no. 4 (2017): 9.
14 Marc Bekoff and Jessica Pierce, *Wild Justice: The Moral Lives of Animals* (Chicago: University of Chicago Press, 2009), 68.
15 Lacan, *Écrits*, 78.
16 Clive D. L. Wynne and Monique A. R. Udell, *Animal Cognition: Evolution, Behavior and Cognition*, 2nd ed. (New York: Palgrave Macmillan, 2013), 173.
17 Martin Heidegger, *Being and Time*, trans. John Macquarrie and Edward Robinson (New York: Harper & Row, 1962).
18 Zwart, "Conditioned Reflexes and the Symbolic Order," 7.
19 Lacan, *Écrits*, 78.
20 Lacan, *Écrits*, 78.
21 Derrida, *The Animal That Therefore I Am*, 12.
22 Derrida, *The Animal That Therefore I Am*, 11.
23 Philip Armstrong, "The Gaze of Animals," in *Theorizing Animals: Re-Thinking Humanimal Relations*, ed. Nik Taylor and Tania Signal (Leiden: Brill, 2011), 178.
24 Armstrong, "The Gaze of Animals," 178.

25 Armstrong, "The Gaze of Animals," 182.
26 Armstrong, "The Gaze of Animals," 182.
27 Armstrong, "The Gaze of Animals," 192.
28 Armstrong, "The Gaze of Animals," 190.
29 Armstrong, "The Gaze of Animals," 189.
30 Armstrong, "The Gaze of Animals," 189.
31 Nicholas Ray, "The Creature Was a Man! Psychoanalysis, Freud, and Animals," in *The Bloomsbury Handbook to Psychoanalysis & Literature*, ed. Jeremy Tambling (London: Bloomsbury, 2022), 409.
32 Ray, "The Creature Was a MAN!" 409.
33 Ray, "The Creature Was a MAN!" 409.
34 Armstrong, "The Gaze of Animals," 189.
35 Melanie Klein, "Mourning and Its Relation to Manic-Depressive States," in *Selected Melanie Klein*, ed. Juliet Mitchell (New York: Simon and Schuster, 1987), 167.
36 Klein, "Mourning and Its Relation to Manic-Depressive States," 168.
37 Klein, "Mourning and Its Relation to Manic-Depressive States," 168.
38 Klein, "Mourning and Its Relation to Manic-Depressive States," 169.
39 Armstrong, "The Gaze of Animals," 197.
40 Lacan, *Four Fundamental Concepts*, 72.
41 Lacan, *Four Fundamental Concepts*, 74.
42 Lacan, *Four Fundamental Concepts*, 83.
43 Lacan, *Four Fundamental Concepts*, 74.
44 Lacan, *Four Fundamental Concepts*, 74.
45 Lacan, *Four Fundamental Concepts*, 75.
46 Lacan, *Four Fundamental Concepts*, 99.
47 Lacan, *Four Fundamental Concepts*, 109.
48 Lacan, *Four Fundamental Concepts*, 89.
49 Lacan, *Four Fundamental Concepts*, 101.
50 Lacan, *Four Fundamental Concepts*, 101.
51 Lacan, *Four Fundamental Concepts*, 101.
52 Lacan, *Four Fundamental Concepts*, 99.
53 Lacan, *Four Fundamental Concepts*, 100.
54 Roger Caillois, "Mimicry and Legendary Psychasthenia," trans. John Shepley, *October* 31 (1984): 17.
55 Caillois, "Mimicry and Legendary Psychasthenia," 22.
56 Caillois, "Mimicry and Legendary Psychasthenia," 23.
57 Caillois, "Mimicry and Legendary Psychasthenia," 25.
58 Caillois, "Mimicry and Legendary Psychasthenia," 30.
59 Caillois, "Mimicry and Legendary Psychasthenia," 28.
60 Caillois, "Mimicry and Legendary Psychasthenia," 32.
61 Sigmund Freud, *Beyond the Pleasure Principle*, trans. James Strachey (New York: W. W. Norton & Company, 1961), 32.
62 Freud, *Beyond the Pleasure Principle*, 30.
63 Freud, *Beyond the Pleasure Principle*, 33.
64 Freud, *Beyond the Pleasure Principle*, 33.
65 Freud, *Beyond the Pleasure Principle*, 43.
66 James Mallet, "Mimicry: An Interface between Psychology and Evolution," *Proceedings of the National Academy of Sciences* 98, no. 16 (2001): 8928.
67 David W. Kikuchi and David W. Pfennig, "Imperfect Mimicry and the Limits of Natural Selection," *The Quarterly Review of Biology* 88, no. 4 (2013): 297.
68 Kikuchi and Pfennig, "Imperfect Mimicry and the Limits of Natural Selection," 297.
69 Kikuchi and Pfennig, "Imperfect Mimicry and the Limits of Natural Selection," 299.
70 Lacan, *Four Fundamental Concepts*, 81.

71 Lacan, *Four Fundamental Concepts*, 84.
72 Jacques Lacan, *My Teaching*, trans. David Macey (London: Verso, 2008), 37.
73 Lacan, *My Teaching*, 37.
74 Lacan, *Écrits*, 720.
75 Jacques-Alain Miller, *Paradigms of Jouissance* (London Society of the New Lacanian School, 2019), 19.
76 Jacques Lacan, *The Formations of the Unconscious: The Seminar of Jacques Lacan, Book V*, ed. Jacques-Alain Miller, trans. Russell Grigg (Cambridge: Polity Press, 2017), 320.
77 Lacan, *Formations of the Unconscious*, 320.
78 Lacan, *Four Fundamental Concepts*, 107.
79 Jacques Lacan, *Anxiety: The Seminar of Jacques Lacan, Book X*, trans. A. R. Price (Cambridge: Polity Press, 2014), 45.
80 Michael F. Land, *Eyes to See: The Astonishing Variety of Vision in Nature* (Oxford: Oxford University Press, 2014), 169.
81 Lacan, *Écrits*, 239.
82 Land, *Eyes to See*, 177.
83 Leonard Harrison Matthews, "Visual Stimulation and Ovulation in Pigeons," *Proceedings of the Royal Society of London B* 126, no. 845 (1939): 557.
84 Matthews, "Visual Stimulation and Ovulation in Pigeons," 559.
85 Wynne and Udell, *Animal Cognition*, 28.
86 John Bowlby, *Attachment*, Vol. 1 of *Attachment and Loss* (New York: Basic Books, 1969), 181.
87 Bowlby, *Attachment*, 181.
88 Bowlby, *Attachment*, 181.
89 Lacan, *Four Fundamental Concepts*, 75.
90 Lacan, *Four Fundamental Concepts*, 83.
91 Lacan, *Four Fundamental Concepts*, 99.
92 Lacan, *Four Fundamental Concepts*, 84.
93 Lacan, *Four Fundamental Concepts*, 84.
94 Lacan, *Four Fundamental Concepts*, 75.
95 Lacan, *Four Fundamental Concepts*, 84.
96 Lacan, *Four Fundamental Concepts*, 74.
97 Lacan, *Four Fundamental Concepts*, 84.
98 Lacan, *Four Fundamental Concepts*, 84.
99 Bruce Fink, *Lacan on Love: An Exploration of Lacan's Seminar VIII, Transference* (Cambridge: Polity Press, 2016), 62.
100 Fink, *Lacan on Love*, 66.
101 Fink, *Lacan on Love*, 68.
102 Fink, *Lacan on Love*, 68.
103 Fink, *Lacan on Love*, 71.
104 Fink, *Lacan on Love*, 71.
105 Fink, *Lacan on Love*, 74.
106 Fink, *Lacan on Love*, 75.
107 Lacan, *Anxiety*, 58.
108 Wynne and Udell, *Animal Cognition*, 182.
109 Lacan, *Écrits*, 400.
110 Fink, *Lacan on Love*, 75.

Chapter 3

Lacan's Praying Mantis

Trauma, Jouissance, and Animality in the Real

If one were to classify animals according to the three psychoanalytic symptomological categories (neurotic, perverse, and psychotic)—animals would undoubtedly be placed under the heading of the psychotic. The psychotic status of animality is unequivocal if considered, at the start, in the negative, since the neurotic and perverted positions are constituted by language (they are both entangled, in singular ways, with the function of the signifier); animals *cannot* be neurotic nor perverse due to a subjective non-relation to the symbolic. Approached positively, animal behavior (if unobstructed by human anthropomorphological preconceptions) is clearly psychotic in their unrestrained, fragmented reality. I consign animals a psychotic status not in order to invent a formal and authentically clinical symptomatology of animality—it does not seem apparent, at this juncture, what an animal symptom in the psychoanalytic field (either in a theoretical or clinical dimension) would mean—the insight is unrelated to a presence of symptoms; instead, the essential point is the structure of animal subjectivity and experience.

For Lacan, what does it mean for one to be psychotic? Lacanian nosological classifications align, in many substantive ways, with the Freudian conception—meaning the Lacanian psychotic is overwhelmingly the Freudian psychotic—though there are, of course, certain not entirely insubstantial interventions introduced by Lacan. Simply, there are some notable Lacanian twists to Freud's conception of the psychotic. Both view the psychotic as interpretable (though they may not necessarily indicate that they are treatable, with the psychotic condition largely viewed as symptomatically inflexible)—the psychotic subject is not beyond psychoanalytic interpretation and understanding. However, for Lacan the psychotic holds a special position to language. The psychotic structure is predicated on "foreclosure":

> [psychosis is caused by] "foreclosure" of the signifier. At the point at which the Name-of-the-Father is summoned . . . a pure and simple hole may thus answer in the Other; due to the lack of metaphoric effect, this hole will give rise to a corresponding hole in the place of phallic signification.[1]

For the psychotic, the "Name-of-the-Father" is entirely foreclosed—the psychotic is shut off, at least temporarily, from integrating this signifier. By "lack of

DOI: 10.4324/9781003635383-5

metaphoric effect," Lacan means that the "hole" (in the symbolic field, caused by the missing name-of-the-father) cannot be inscribed by any set of signifiers; there is no 'metaphor' for the name-of-the-father that is foreclosed.

Of course, this signifier represents much more than a single word—and is certainly not synonymous with the literal name of the subject's father; the-name-of-the-father represents the Law itself along with the symbolic apparatus that dispenses this Law: through the foreclosure of the name-of-the-father, the psychotic subject comes to be cut off from the structure of the symbolic universe that characterizes, in the most immediate manner, human society. What is human social organization if not precisely the affiliation based on this symbolic Law (that is foreclosed for the psychotic subject)? In clinical psychoanalysis, the human psychotic subject exhibits symptoms such as disruptions of speech and a distinctly unreal relationship to the external world due to an unmediated, direct confrontation with the Real, caused by the foreclosure of The-Name-Of-The-Father. Psychoanalyst Russell Grigg explains that, according to Lacanian thought, "that which is foreclosed from the symbolic reappears in the real."[2] In psychosis, foreclosure from the symbolic universe results in a reappearance—which haunts the subject in its enigmatic form—from the vantage of the Real, articulated via symbolic means.

In what way is the animal psychotic? They are psychotic precisely because their subjectivity is structurally foreclosed to *even the possibility of any signifier*. Structural foreclosure is, of course, distinct from the human who exists in language yet *loses* or, more aptly, never properly incorporates, the locus of the symbolic into their subjectivity (the symbolic Other). Animals would not display a symptomology—since this is not a loss of something they *should* have (their foreclosure, unlike the human's, is pre-inscribed in their being—they are foreclosed at the ontological level of species). However, we see here that the behavior of animals is naturally psychotic in a non-pathological sense: A psychotic state is the inherent *given* of animal subjectivity. The point here is not to designate a collapse of the human psychotic subject into animality—for the human psychotic, the foreclosure of the name-of-the-father (the structural anchoring point that heralds in Law as such) is a genuine *loss*, in the sense that one is alienated (due to the foreclosure) from the socio-organizational makeup *in which they already exist*. Conversely, for animals, as we have seen, the lack of the signifier of Law does not designate a loss (leading to certain problems with animal-human relations in the domestic sphere—with humans inscribed in Law and animals not).

Animals are largely psychotic in this sense—placing them (almost) squarely in the position of a direct confrontation with the Real. The encounter with the Real is still mediated, through a register which refracts and splinters its unbearability, though in a distinct way from humans. (Crucially, the animal's experience of the Real is mediated through the imaginary register.) Psychosis leads the human subject to directly contend with the Real without the necessary mediator of a symbolic universe bounded together by Law—the Real spills into their reality, resulting in a disrupted, disjointed reality replete with hallucinations and delusions (consider, for instance, the famous case study by Freud of Judge Schreber's memoir, a psychotic judge who experiences distinctly unreal sensations such as immediate contact with God and believing himself to be a messianic, Jesus-like redeemer of humanity); for the animal, the psychotic structure does not lead to these same symptoms (or necessarily any symptoms) because their subjectivity does not rely on the structure of the signifier. Grigg explains this paradoxical tension between the psychotics' delusions (such as Judge Schreber's), that rely on the signifier, and the psychotics' very foreclosure from the symbolic field:

> On the one hand, the content of hallucinations is structured by the symbolic. On the other, because what reappears in hallucinations has been foreclosed from the symbolic, it is simply obvious that it cannot have the structure of the symbolic . . . . Nevertheless, what paranoid psychosis makes apparent, and it is a point that Lacan often repeats, is that the structure of the real is determined by the signifier. This is particularly apparent in discussions of Schreber, where we never encounter the real except as structured by the signifier . . . . These phenomena, which are specific to psychosis, nevertheless remain phenomena of signifiers. In other words, the real of Schreber's hallucinations is structured by the signifier. And this is exactly Lacan's point.[3]

Grigg makes an essential intervention into the discourse on psychosis here: Regardless of being foreclosed to the signifier (in terms of the Law that the signifier brings), the Real that intrudes into the subject (hallucinations, for instance) is structured by the signifier. He calls this a 'symbolized real' and concludes that

> *No encounter with the real that is not mediated by the symbolic is possible in either psychosis or neurosis.* Or, in other words: *Every encounter with the real, whether in neurosis or psychosis, is mediated by the symbolic.*[4]

The signifier, even for one who has not annexed the fabric of the symbolic Law, remains the locus of the Real—as Lacan writes of the "drama of madness": "it is in man's relation to the signifier that this drama is situated."[5] Here, we see the strict demarcation between an animal and human experience of the Real, and why, although animals can nominally be called psychotic, they do not have the same pathological effects or symptoms that the human experiences: Since the human has already entered into the symbolic universe (they participate in speech) even their experience of the Real is refracted (nonsensically and unrecognizably for others, since it is unbound by a unifying symbolic system) through the signifier. Simply, even the psychotic's subjectivity is structured by the signifier (despite the foreclosure of the signifier's Law) which is why the intrusion of the Real has such troubling effects: *The Real meets a symbolic un-structured by a Law, due to the foreclosure of the vital Name-of-the-Father signifier and its paternal function*—there is no structural Law to restrain this reappearance, and the Real then dramatically erupts in all its abrasive, nonsensical nature through the symbolic.

In animality, we see no such symptoms because the tension between the implicitly present signifier and the foreclosure from the symbolic field does not exist—there is no such thing as a symbolized Real for the animal. Instead, the imaginary acts as the structural anchoring point that binds their subjective planes. This insight into the mediating distance of the imaginary distinguishes our approach from the banal criticism, deployed against Lacan, that he relegates animals to an inaccessible Real, forever epistemically precluding the human from knowing the animal. As the foregoing chapters have shown, animal interiority can be retrieved from its putative vacantness despite animals' lack of signifier use—and, as we will now see, also despite their proximity to the Real. Human psychosis, and the animal's analogous position as asymptomatically psychotic, offers a plain insight into the subjectivity of animality: If the psychotic human can be epistemically accessed through psychoanalytic theory (and, of course, clinical practice), through their continued reliance on the structure of the signifier, then the animal can be known, in their relation to the Real, through the structure of the imaginary. The animal and the Real (that both act as sites of radical discontinuity, defying formulization and the symbolic) are not entirely sealed off from theoretical psychoanalytical knowledge.

The Traumatic Real and Animality

Trauma—an arresting disjuncture piercing reality, encountered by both humans and animals—is a useful conceptual entry-point to explicate the Real and its bearing on animality. Freud articulates trauma as an economic deluge of stimulus that subsumes the subject's defenses: "We describe as 'traumatic' any excitations from outside which are powerful enough to break through the protective shield."[6] Lacan, through his development of the Real register, names the field outside of powerful "excitations" and provides a topological theory of what exactly is 'broken through.' Considering the Real in its traumatic dimension, as humans experience it, offers an unambiguous definition: the traumatic Real is that which is unsymbolizable; it is precisely those encounters that cannot capitulate to the signifier. The Real, as Lacan (uncharacteristically) straightforwardly declares, is the "domain of that which subsists outside of symbolization."[7] To Lacan, the Real is "the impossible"[8] and, as he says elsewhere, it is the "limit" of the subject's self-understanding or of the subject's "recalling of his biography."[9] In Lacanian thought, the Real cannot be submitted to the order of the signifier—there is always some remainder that is 'unassimilable,' and this remainder is located exactly where the Real, in its traumatic character, crashes into the symbolic universe of the subject. Trauma is experienced in all its radicality, its utter alterity from our day-to-day existence, due to its supralinguistic Real nature: trauma is traumatic because of its non-relation to language and inability (at some level) to undergo significantization. However, despite this resistance, the signifier is pre-determinative of the Real's re-appearance in human subjectivity.

The necessary distinction, in order for the Real to not be viewed as a purely semantic Francophone play on reality or the Kantian noumenon (the 'thing-in-itself'), is this: while reality, as defined in the human sphere of experientiality, is organized by the linguistic field (the symbolic and the Signifier), the Real is precisely the un-linguistifizable elements of experience that pierce reality. If reality is that which can be understood and is organized by the symbolic register, then the Real is the presence of an unreality that exceeds the symbolic. Lacan explains that the Real is "ready to submerge with its roar what the 'reality principle' constructs there that goes by the name of the 'outside world.'"[10] Here, we see that the Real cannot be collapsed into an empirical externality: Lacan directly opposes the Real and the "outside world." Yet, stopping there would appear to enable a conflation of the Real and the Kantian noumenon: *Isn't the Real merely the kernel of objects that forever resists symbolization and comprehension, the unknowable inner-being of the world that somehow slams into our symbolic-based reality?* The Kantian noumenon, of course, could be considered traumatic given its enigmatic unknowability—however, the Real is not something that 'is' traumatic (the externalized event) but is instead what gives trauma its character in the traumatized recipient (it is trauma itself). To be clear here: Though the Real always, at least partially, remains inarticulable and fundamentally resistant to linguistic efforts, it becomes traumatic through introducing a hole *from within* the symbolic universe. The traumatic Real enters into language and, through this collision with the symbolic, becomes known in its inaccessibility to the signifier—which language then proceeds to circle around impotently. This is why Lacan refers to the Real as "that which always comes back to the same place"[11]—the Real remains occluded in language while the signifier continually returns to the Real in the attempt to articulate it (the Real remains immovable despite the language applied to it in discourse: the Real is a stone which can be painted by words but never truly effaced). The traumatic is the unsaid—the unsaid that remains sealed off from language as Real, the very limit of signification and the entire symbolic field.

We must also consider here the private status of the Real, particularly in its traumatic dimension: The Real is only known in proximity to an individuated psychicality—the Real could not be constituted as such purely as an externalized existent. Simply, the encounter with the Real is a private event. Embedded in the Real is a facticity external to the subject (the Real *is* something from *outside* subjectivity but also *within* the symbolic field); however, the Real is only known via its intrusion into subjectivity, colliding into the symbolic and reaching the subject's consciousness. This is the crucial difference: Everything, in its facticity, exists outside the symbolic register and, in the Kantian sense, resists symbolization and a finality of understanding (this is the basic insight into the function of the signifier: it holds an arbitrary relation to the signified along with the referent supposedly 'behind' the signified, and accordingly everything that is empirical cannot be submitted through language; the world exceeds language)—but everything that exists is certainly not traumatic. There always exists a severance, a fundamentally untraversable partitional gap between language and the objective, non-symbolically mediated world—however, an event only takes on a traumatic character in relation to an individuated subjectivity (albeit, of course, an event can be intersubjectively traumatic in the sense of being traumatic across a number of subjectivities, such as 9/11).

An encounter is traumatic insofar as it remains a point of occlusion in the subject's symbolic universe. In a sense, the Real is negatively present (present as an absence of symbolization)—as the gap in the symbolic itself, rather than the actual event in its facticity and objective nature. Žižek corroborates this distinction between the Real and reality, describing it as such:

> reality . . . serves as the external boundary which enables us to totalize language, to make out of it a close and coherent system, whereas the Real is its inherent limit, the unfathomable fold which prevents it from achieving its identity with itself.[12]

Žižek ascribes to reality a function as an "external boundary" that grants our language a symbolic coherence—and is this not precisely the meaning we assign to reality in our everyday relations? Our common, everyday phrases denote this same meaning: *They need to get a grip on reality* or *They are crazy—they need a reality check.* These phrases function to designate reality as the consistent, ever-reliable anchoring point that generates a "close and coherent system" that one must, according to the latent meaning of these phrases, return to in order to make sense of our lives.

The Real, inversely, is the "unfathomable" that does not pierce from *without* but, instead, punctures from *within* reality and the symbolic field, acting as an "inherent limit" to their coherence and preventing, interminably, a fully integrated self-same identity with itself—the Real contests the coherence of reality, injecting a site of utter heterogeneity that forever resists symbolization. The problem, paradoxically, is not the signifiers' 'impossibility to touch the Real,' but instead the symbolics' inherent impossibility of ever fully attaining itself—the lack of a closed, coherent totality in the symbolic is what permits the crisis of the Real to emerge. This lack, endemic to language, results in an object which "inscribes itself in the blank opened by this failure."[13] The crisis of failure implicit in the symbolic is precisely the point the Real comes to occupy—and we see here why an object from 'reality' brings comfort while an object that occupies the site of the Real brings terror, since it exhibits, sometimes viscerally, the lack inherent to our symbolic universe.

To take a straightforward instance: A sexual act always exceeds language in its objective facticity—one can refer to it as 'making love' or 'intercourse' or be hyper-descriptive and apply a lengthy string of signifiers attempting to capitulate the act to language, but the act can never be totally captured or articulated in speech. One does not normally encounter psychic pain associated with this inability to articulate the act—the lack inherent to language is not apparent to the subject (albeit there is certainly an element of sexuality that is Real, namely jouissance, which can present its own symptoms—and some subjects may be haunted by the lack inherent to language itself, feeling eternally alienated from others); the conventional sexual act is not ordinarily traumatic: Intercourse takes on a traumatic feature only when it presents a disjuncture in the symbolic network, introducing a pronounced gap that cannot be registered (such as sexual abuse). Because one is able to register, or index, an 'ordinary' sexual act (despite the severance between sexuality, in terms of its physical activity, and language) it is precluded from gaining a traumatic status for the subject (the sexual act burrows within the symbolic field, averting it from remaining heterogenous from language itself)—and when one is not able to index the act into their symbolic network, the severance between the act and language is rendered explicit and introduces a gap which language circles, again and again, seeking to fill a negative site. One should observe here that, while there are empirical events (acts of violence, injuries—both psychic and physical—and encounters with death or loss) that are widely detected as 'traumatic,' the Real does not exist *out there* in the objective encounter but rather exists *within* the subject *through* the encounter. It is a negative encounter in the symbolic network with that which cannot be articulated or properly indexed and consequently repeats itself through the signifier's return to its inexplicable gap-site.

This is why an event can appear un-traumatic, in the objective sense, while holding a traumatic status for the subject—it is the relation to subjectivity and their symbolic network that renders it a traumatic Real. To provide a somewhat stale, stereotypical example, consider fireworks for the veteran with PTSD: The fireworks themselves hold nothing traumatic in their 'objective' facticity, but the encounter nonetheless can introduce an unsymbolizable site of a traumatic Real. The fireworks, while always exceeding language, act as a reminder of an earlier, originary Real (presumably the war, with its bombs and gunshots) retained in the subject. In this case, though, the fireworks may later be indexed, or partially dissolved (*it was only fireworks, I am okay*), but the Real of war that the fireworks momentarily represented or were the causation of a traumatic return remains—with language failing to fill it in, since one cannot fully submit the traumatic experience of war to signification.

This precise function of the intrusion of a traumatic Real is found in the 2009 film *Brothers*. After returning from Afghanistan, Sam Cahill (played by Toby Maguire), is sitting at the dinner table with his family—and during this tense dinner, two events from reality occur that precipitate an aggressive reaction indicative of PTSD (culminating in Cahill yelling and striking across the table at his daughter's balloon): The first, a semantically direct reference to the site of his traumatic Real, is his young daughter's mention of the word "Afghanistan" ("I didn't get anything I wanted for my birthday—and you were in stupid Afghanistan")[14] and the second is a more innocuous gesture in which his daughter rubs a balloon between her hands, which possibly, for Cahill, subtly mimics the sound of distant gunfire. Here, we come to an insight acting in full obviosity: These gestures by the daughter, while equally apparent in their status in *reality* (meaning all present at the table can perceive the comment on Afghanistan and hear the noise of the balloon), have a particular impression on Cahill as a recipient since, for him, these are vestiges of the Real and consequently prompt a PTSD-informed outburst. This scene perfectly articulates the gulf between the Real and reality as such; it is not about the Real that purely exists out there in reality, but rather a relation between something (whether it exists in reality or not) and a particular psychic interiority.

Žižek supplies an instructive example of the Real that designates its place in language and relation to trauma:

> trauma is *real*—it is a hard core resisting symbolization, but the point is that it does not matter if it has had a place, if it has 'really occurred' in so called reality . . . . The most famous Freudian example of such a real entity is of course the primal parricide: it would be senseless to search for its traces in prehistoric reality, but it must none the less be presupposed if we want to account for the present state of things . . . . The paradox of the Lacanian Real, then, is that it is an entity which, although it does not exist (in the sense of 'really existing', taking place in reality), has a series of properties—it exercises a certain structural causality, it can produce a series of effects in the symbolic reality of subjects.[15]

Freud's primal horde, referring, of course, to the postulated historical parricide by a band of brothers which inaugurates the Oedipus complex, is a traumatic Real regardless of its historicity: it does not matter if one cannot locate this event in "prehistorical reality" since its effects account "for the present state of things." The traumatic Real does not necessarily exist in facticity as long as it generates "a series of effects" in the subject—a manufactured or fantasized Real, that one believes occurred, could have the same effects. We should observe here, though, that the Real is not necessarily something that is fictitious or totally severed from external reality—there are certainly traumatic points that properly exist in reality, but the crucial insight here is that the mere existence in the 'out there' of reality is not what renders it traumatic.

As defined so far, the Real has only been conceived of in its relation to the symbolic. Largely, for Lacan, this is how the Real, at least in its traumatic dimension, is understood—as an intrusion upon the symbolic that is circled by language. In this conception, the Real has no true bearing on animality due to the primacy of the imaginary, rather than the symbolic, in their subjectivity. How, then, does the veridicality of animal trauma maintain its position as undeniable? As I will exhibit shortly, the research on animal trauma affirms its existence—functioning like human trauma but independent of the symbolic field. The facticity of animal trauma means that the traumatic Real must puncture the imaginary field that organizes the reality of animals. When an animal experiences trauma, they experience an event that cannot be submitted to the visual-scopic (imaginary) field—and, like the human, the traumatic Real inexorably emerges from the encounter with an individuated subjectivity that cannot be indexed. Further—just like the human who fails to incorporate a traumatic Real into their symbolic network, forcing a negative severance that makes itself apparent through the repeating failures of language to designate the Real's (symbolic) hollow space, resulting in a perpetual return the animal's experience of the traumatic Real is of an analogous return, caused by the failure of the imaginary network.

Animal trauma is seen along the same lines as the human experience of trauma: a piercing that cannot be incorporated into their (in this case, imaginary) universe. While one could attempt to put this in purely physiological terms—rendering any event traumatic which applies a sufficient shock to the central nervous system, being unincorporated in the physical, sensory sense, rather than turning to interiority and animal subjectivity—a positivist conception of trauma (which, as we will see, many animal researchers mechanistically rely on, appealing almost entirely to neurological explanations) fails to account for aspects of animal trauma that remain unexplored.

Eslom's Trauma: The Real Overtaking the Imaginary

I will begin the discussion of animal trauma in familiar mammalian-primate territory: the chimpanzee. Animal researchers in the article "Signs of Mood and Anxiety Disorders in Chimpanzees," write that, "[c]omplex PTSD, depression, and other psychiatric conditions have been diagnosed in other species [than humans], including chimpanzees."[16] The researchers collected published case reports of chimpanzees in both the wild and "currently living in sanctuaries as a result of previous use in laboratory research, illegal trade and seizure, or being orphaned" and developed criteria—consisting of a "cluster of symptoms" based on "the criteria for PTSD and depression listed in the DSM-IV."[17] Then, they deployed these criteria to assess chimpanzees for comparable trauma-induced PTSD and depression, concluding: "previously traumatized chimpanzees demonstrate persistent abnormal objective symptoms and that these symptoms cluster into syndromes that are similar to PTSD and depression."[18] Although the diagnostic criteria for human PTSD/depression and chimpanzee PTSD/depression are not indistinguishable (meaning the criteria for humans are not directly superimposed onto the criteria for animals)—largely due to the languagelessness of chimpanzees, leading the researchers to rely on a diagnostic criteria drawn from the "alternative criteria" used for "PTSD in nonverbal infants and children"[19]—it remains clear that the presence of these symptomatic clusters signify an *equivalent* condition in chimpanzees, and that these conditions originate from a site (or multiple sites) of trauma.

In the article, the researchers supply instructive 'case vignettes' from the chimpanzees, describing the traumatic instances and the subsequently developed symptomatic behavior, causally linking them. The cases begin with a chimpanzee named Negra who was "taken from the wild in Africa as an infant" and subsequently "remained in captivity," meeting the alternative criteria for "depression and PTSD."[20] When she was initially captured, Negra was used for "invasive research" and was kept isolated from other chimpanzees. After being brought to a sanctuary with six other chimpanzees, she exhibited symptoms that aligned with a traumatic encounter, such as "persistent depressed hunched posture" and being "socially withdrawn."[21] Additionally, "caretakers reported that her face was expressionless, 'like a ghost,' for at least a month after she arrived at the sanctuary."[22] All these behaviors are indicative of the long-term effects of trauma: Events in Negra's life have left her with a sustained traumatic impression in her subjectivity. One should recall that, in Lacanian terms, trauma is "that which always comes back to the same place," perpetually returning despite its temporal position as already occurred. They are fragments from the past that haunt the present—it is a site of the traumatic Real. Is this not precisely what Negras experiences when a traumatic past haunts her present?

Another chimpanzee, named Eslom, was tracked by researchers in the wild with a group of other chimpanzees, and for him, there are a series of early familial tragedies: At the age of 13, his mother died—then, a few years later, his younger sister "who exhibited ongoing behavioral effects from being orphaned at a young age"[23] disappeared from his primate group. Eslom also endured physical trauma after being trapped in a 'snare' while in the wild, with no sustained injury or disabilities caused by the snare incident. After these patently traumatic incidents,

> Eslom exhibited several ongoing behaviors consistent with the alternative criteria for PTSD . . . . He remained aroused [in terms of aggression] for unusually long periods of time, and it took him a long time for him [sic] to calm down after incidents . . . . Avoidance and fear behaviors were reported, along with social withdrawal.[24]

These aberrative, non-normative behaviors classify Eslom squarely as experiencing PTSD—as a being who has, after undergoing some traumatic event, sustained effects prolonged across their lifetime (or for a significant portion of their life).

When converted to the Lacanian lexicon, we see an encounter with the Real is the originary cause for Eslom's PTSD-adjacent symptoms. What are these sustained effects (social isolation, recurring fear, aggression) if not the compulsory 'repeating' following the Real's collision with the structural constitution of Eslom's subjectivity? A traumatic event, for the chimpanzee, is precisely an encounter that defies the 'reality' constituted by the chimpanzee's imaginary subjectivity. Eslom's experiences—the loss of his mother and later his sister, dissolved his familial organization. It would be said, for a human, to be 'beyond words.' These traumatic sites, in human subjectivity, would be rendered traumatic for their extra-linguistic nature: the excessiveness of an event—its non-submission to symbolization (as Lacan says, the traumatic Real is 'unassimilable' to the symbolic)—is the defining mark of the Real to the human. For the animal, though, the excessiveness of an event is not inscribed as traumatic due to its non-submission to the symbolic—but instead due to its non-submission to the imaginary dimension.

In what way is Eslom's imaginary constitution of subjectivity punctured by the loss of his mother and sister? It is crucial to observe that Eslom's posttraumatic disorder is not solely brought on by being subjected to physical pain—while the snare is cited and certainly contributed towards Eslom's condition, it is not the isolated traumatic instance that led to his cluster of PTSD-like symptoms. Extreme pain is undoubtedly traumatic (and the trauma of pain in animality will be explored later), but for Eslom there is concurrently a social dimension to his suffering: the death of his mother and disappearance of his sister threaten the social order which constitutes Eslom as himself in the imaginary domain. As John Bowlby delineates, the attachment between a chimpanzee and their mother is indisputable: "the baby chimpanzee spends the whole of its infancy in close proximity to its mother. During the first four months it clings to her in the ventral position and only very occasionally is seen apart from here."[25] And this attachment does not end in adolescence: "up to the time of reaching puberty [chimpanzee] males were still spending at least half their time with mother; and each of them continued to meet his mother occasionally up to the time of her death."[26] There is an attachment here that cannot be easily dismissed—one that exceeds nourishing a baby. Loss of the object of that attachment (the mother) is plainly traumatic because it punctures Eslom's own imaginary self-hood.

This point should not be confused by anthropocentric superimposition: It is not the 'I' (enacted in language through enunciation) that is threatened, nor is the self-signifier 'Eslom' under attack, since no symbolic designation exists and therefore cannot be lost—but rather the imaginary, non-lingual sense of self that Eslom possesses is what comes under attack. With the loss of the parent and the sibling, Eslom feels that *he* is what is lost. The imaginary conception of self—an image of self—is predicated on the image of another: Eslom, however he conceives of himself, is constituted by the identification-image (the sensory presence) of his family, and an absence of this (visual-tactile-auditory-olfactory) image is an absence of his conception of self.

Critically, we can detect here a residue of the Real: As established, the Real is not something entirely externally imposed (an encounter with the forever-unknown Kantian noumenon-thing is not what spurs the traumatic response) since the Real emerges from within the very field it penetrates. As we noted in the instance of humans, the Real is concomitant with the symbolic, forcing open a crevice from within the symbolic field and bringing awareness to a pronounced gap. In short, the traumatic Real, for animals, is not an intrusion totally extrinsic to the imaginary dimension; the Real is, instead, a gap within the imaginary field. Of course, Elsom's mother dying and sister disappearing are both extra-subjective events transpiring in the 'reality' of the world 'out there'—they are external events which transcend his interiority (a simple point: these events are irreducible to his experience of them; they have an unequivocal veridicality). Instead, the events are traumatic because they draw attention to the bounds of the imaginary field: For the chimpanzee, a loss of family undermines the attempts for their imaginary network to bind the Real—the failure of the imaginary (the relative impotence of the scopic domain to structure subjectivity without permitting holes, whether those be of self-image or image-of-others) to designate some external event in reality is precisely what generates the traumatic Real. There is no longer the imaginary barrier against the Real—only a failure experienced as Real.

Simply, in the case of Eslom, he was always a subjectivity isolated from other subjectivities—an island of interiority (though one that is developmentally interdependent—formed by others and the Other)—and the loss of those who define this self-image (the sister and the mother) results in a confrontation with this alienating cavity in the imaginary structure. As Lacan claims, the imaginary and its identifications, like the symbolic universe, always lead to an "alienating destination."[27] Although animals certainly have a closer proximal immanence to their bodies—comparatively less severed, when compared to humans, due to the lack of symbolic—there is still the gap that imaginary identifications introduce. If we brought the imaginary scene into language, these identifications for a being such as Eslom appear in the form of: *That is a being like me/That is a being not like me* (species identification upon seeing another chimpanzee or seeing another species unlike his own); *That being is me* (bodily self-consciousness upon seeing himself, for instance in a mirror); *I am not me without that being* (immediate familial identification upon seeing those that constitute his closest community-unit). The latter is precisely why Eslom losing his mother has an incongruous impact when compared to a different form of identification with the dead, such as encountering a dead corpse of an unknown chimpanzee in the forest (an identification with death-loss on the plane of species). His mother was a constitutive part of himself on the imaginary plane. The unknown corpse does not occupy the same imaginary position as the dead family member.

We should not appear to falsely attribute a sense of death to animality. Animals have a sense of loss without a sense of death. Animals do not apprehend death and the finitude of life or temporality—they do not understand what Heidegger calls the 'horizon of life,' which is the ever-present prospect of dying, the terminating site of life in every direction (its 'horizon') that delimits life as self-contained. But animals do sense the absence of an attachment-object. Eslom does not apprehend the fact that his mother will never return—she is dead in all of death's finality—but he undoubtedly apprehends the fact of her absence in a given moment, and the accumulation of those moments has an emotional force. There is a tacit understanding (of loss) without a conceptual or representational understanding (of death). An instructive example: I witnessed, after one of my mother-in-law's dogs died, another of her dogs approach the corpse, brushing his nose against the body to re-animate it. After repeated attempts, the dog began howling in what I would classify (despite the risk of anthropomorphization) as a howl of mourning, where the dog registered another subject as absent—the body of the dog's companion was present, but his animating force, his inner-being (denoted, perceptually, by movement), was utterly absent. The dog knew nothing of death yet recognized loss and non-presence in presence—an image of the other was shattered by the imposition of the Real. What could this loss be, for the living dog, if not a constitutive element of himself, through the absence of an-other who he spent years beside? The animal's pain of loss is an analog to the human's pain of loss-via-death, both dealing with identifications with the other. What is lost, for both the human and the animal, is not only the other but the imaginary sense of oneself.

It is essential to note here that these effects of the traumatic Real in the social dimension are absolutely not isolated to chimpanzees or dogs. The dreams (or nightmares) of tortured rats operate according to the same principle of a return of the Real: David Peña-Guzman writes that after a group of rats was "physically tortured with shocks to the feet," they began to display "total freezing behavior"[28] (a response indicative of PTSD) when re-introduced to the same enclosure where they were exposed to the shocks. Subsequently, their sleep activity was assessed in the enclosure, and the rats had brain activity which "demonstrated that the rats were experiencing nightmares triggered by traumatic memories."[29] Further, another study on rat sleep-activity, monitoring rats navigating a track while awake, found that, when asleep, the rats occupied a dream-world that reflected "the spatial test they had just completed."[30] In other words, they dreamed of an "internal simulation . . . the rats were dreaming of running the track."[31] Taken together, this means that the rat nightmares of the shocks were a spatial re-capitulation of their torture, a return of the Real in the register of the imaginary—the nightmares were attempts by the rat's imaginary structure to capture the elusive *beyond* of the torturous Real they were subjected to. Further, and essential to understanding the Real in its traumatic dimension, the scene of torture remains unexhausted by the rat's imaginary attempting to apprehend it through pictorial-sensational representation: The torture is a site of the traumatic Real for the rat precisely due to the failure of the imaginary to account for its traumatic content, compelling the rat's subjectivity (structured by the imaginary) to perpetually return to the aperture of the Real.

Elephants exhibit a capacity for social loss similar to the chimpanzees from the case studies, indicating an analogous PTSD-like set of behaviors. In an article published in *Frontiers in Zoology* by mammalian cognition scholar Graeme Shannon and other researchers, they studied the long-term, persistent effects of 'culling' (the purposive reduction of a wildlife population by selective slaughter) on elephants. Like the research on chimpanzee PTSD, elephants who experienced a loss of a family member, or separation from their social unit, had persistent effects of that act as long-term behavioral consequences of traumatic (namely socially disruptive) incidents. As Shannon et al. explain:

> extremely disruptive events, including culling, poaching and translocation to new areas or capture for captivity can ultimately lead to serious disruptions of the intricate social networks that underpin social structure in these species [such as elephants], with severe impacts on each individual's close social bonds.[32]

After analyzing the behavior of elephants who had experienced a traumatic, socially disruptive event (usually separating them from their kin-relations), the researchers discovered that "such disruption appears capable of driving aberrant behaviors in social animals that are akin to the post-traumatic stress disorder experienced by humans following extremely traumatic events."[33] Specifically, the "abnormal social structure" that elephants are left with after "anthropogenic disturbance" can lead to "significantly altered"[34] decision-making skills. For instance, the researchers discovered that a set of elephants who had experienced a familial trauma had comparatively diminished "social discrimination abilities."[35] They were unable to discern if a 'caller' (the sound issued from another elephant) presented a greater threat based on available sensory information (primarily audio-olfactory). In short, their survival instincts are impeded due to the traumatic instance.

The researchers attribute these effects to a lack of "knowledge transfer"[36] due to loss of older kin. Simply, the younger elephants do not have the opportunity to learn from the older elephants, stunting their capacity to discern prospective threats in the calls issued from other elephants. While this offers a partial answer to the elephants' lacking decision-making skills—the researchers subsequently offer another response that places the experiences of elephants precisely in the domain of the traumatic Real (and this response appears to have greater explanatory power): the diminished skills are also due to "neurological changes" that occur in the "large hippocampus of the African elephants."[37] The stunted survival capacities are due not only to a lack of knowledge transfer caused by an irregular social structure, but also to stunted hippocampal development. The hippocampus, as the locus of memory, learning, and emotional regulation in mammalian vertebrate species, can be damaged by a traumatic event. A traumatic episode—such as an elephant witnessing the death of their family members (father, mother, siblings)—especially if experienced during adolescence, when the hippocampus is still developing, could elicit "neurological changes" that preclude the elephant from establishing normative learning and decision-making skills, forever altering their social behavior.

Research on elephant trauma presents an insightful overlap with the article on chimpanzees, which also attributed the non-normative behavior of chimpanzees such as Negra and Eslom to hippocampal activity and development. The researchers write that,

> In humans PTSD has been associated with reductions in hippocampal volume or activity, perhaps because of recurrently and chronically elevated levels of cortisol, followed by down-regulation of the hypothalamic-pituitary-adrenal axis. Abnormalities of this axis have been described in animals subjected to confinement, restraint, isolation, or surgical procedures.[38]

This reduction in hippocampal "volume or activity"—which they unequivocally connect to human PTSD and more tentatively connect to animal PTSD—is the sole reason (neurological or otherwise) they cite for the chimpanzee's experience of trauma.

An article on the trauma of wild animals similarly relies on a neurological answer to animal trauma. After determining that predatorial-induced fear (invoked by a "natural cue" of predator presence such as vocalization) can lead to PTSD-like behavioral changes in wild animals (namely free-living chickadees in this particular study), the researchers link fear-induced "enduring effects on the amygdala and hippocampus"[39] to the long-term behavior changes that are analogous to human PTSD symptoms. The study deliberately engendered a traumatic reaction in the chickadees by housing them in isolated chambers and exposing them for "2 days to audio playbacks of the vocalizations of either predators (treatment group) or non-predators (control group)."[40] The researchers then discovered the sustained effects on behaviors and corresponding neurological activity. After euthanizing the birds (a cruel end to an already cruel experiment), researchers found evidence of a surplus of activity in the amygdala—responsible, for avian species as well as mammals, for "fear processing and the acquisition and expression of fear memories"[41]—and neuronal activity in the hippocampus also associated with trauma. Accordingly, the researchers conclude that the audio playback resulted in immediate neuronal activity that caused non-normative behaviors. Like the other studies, the neurological element is identified as the locus of animal trauma—this means that the animal experiences of trauma, from chimpanzees to elephants and birds, are all neurological reactions to an overwhelming sensory stimulus.

However, we must ask ourselves: Do neurological alterations to regions of the brain such as the hippocampus and amygdala offer a comprehensive explanation of subjective trauma? What is left out by a purely materialist-neurological response to the question of trauma (whether on the plane of humanity or animality)? Is there not an inner-animal subjectivity that eludes the image that a brain scan presents? Here, we confront a fortified bias in the 'scientific' conception of animal (and, increasingly, also human) subjectivity: The territory of the subjective is frequently ceded to the privileged, putatively hyper-objective space of the neurological—as if neurology exhausts the space of interiority and subjectivity. There are philosophical objections that bar a purely neurological response to the question of human subjectivity—but those same objections are not fully erected for the animal, leaving animals relatively defenseless, with only neurological answers to a more diffuse and amorphous question of phenomenological being and subjectivity.

Psychoanalysis and the Real: A Response to the Neurological Explanation of Animal Trauma

Elisabeth Roudinesco, in her scholarly historiographical account of Freud's life, writes that the thesis of psychoanalysis was competing against the unproductive medical nihilism of Freud's time that neglected "subjective suffering, which science had left aside."[42] Psychoanalysis is, of course, the compelling inverse to early-20th-century medical nihilism: A clinical approach centered almost entirely on the articulation of subjective suffering. Putting aside psychic suffering (not in the name of nihilism, but rather to remain epistemically circumscribed by the animal subject), a scientific conception of animality eventually confronts the same problematic as medical nihilism, with the abandonment of animal subjectivity—psychoanalysis (with its centrality of the subject) offers an antidote to the primacy of materialism in approaches such as neurology.

The neurological answer to animal trauma, while accurate in the register of a pure scientism (it is true, of course, that there is a correlative-causal relation between certain neurological activity and specific behaviors, and further that these neuronal alterations are caused by excessive, fear and anxiety-inducing, external sensory stimuli), nonetheless neglects the domain of animal interiority. The animal experience is taken to be a semi-automatic, subject-less 'response' to stimuli—something comparable to a computer keyboard's 'experience' of water producing an electronic malfunction (a computational misfire caused by purely external interference). While the neurological field offers a mechanical answer to animal trauma, it does not offer an individuated, phenomenal account of that trauma—and trauma is indubitably irreducible to neuronal activity, occurring as a recurrent episodic incident in the psychic arena. Animal trauma's phenomenality instead necessitates a psychoanalytic—specifically Lacanian—topology.

A topology of animal trauma, as we will see, is contingent on the fabric of the imaginary and the intrusion of the Real—this does not mean the psychoanalytic approach negates or contradicts the neurological, but it does furnish us with a more supple and intimate understanding of animal interiority transcending analysis on the plane of physicality. Neurology empirically delineates a causal chain that can be narrativized: An incident occurs that is an instantiation of what is received as traumatic for the animal (ranging from a physical injury, to fear of a predator, isolation, or familial loss) and this causes a sustained rise in a physiological fear-response, such as a dramatic rise in cortisol levels (a hormone released by stressful stimuli) that effects the neurological activity in brain regions such as the hippocampus and amygdala. An essential intervention can be made here by the Real: How does an occurrence—which transpires like any other spatiotemporal event—become indexed as traumatic? Why is the loss of Eslom's mother, the elephant whose group has been subjected to poachers, or the rat's torture, registered as a traumatic event? We could appeal here to the neurological or physiological answer: The traumatic event is an 'overwhelming' stimulus that places the animal in a hyper-alarmed state, with the animal's body reflexively responding to an event that could result in the extinguishing of life itself, which goes against the animal's intuitive physiological impulse to sustain life—and results in the enduring effects of trauma, such as the symptomatic cluster of PTSD-like behaviors. However, something crucial is omitted by this, namely: the proper reason why one event, rather than another, is received as traumatic. Yes, an event can be identified as traumatic and its impact located in a region of the brain and even measured—but why is one event an instantiation of trauma over another? To return to the chimpanzee Elsom, a reference to the functioning of the hippocampus does not exhaustively inform us why the death of his mother is qualitatively distinct from encountering any other chimpanzee corpse—both are a confrontation with a no longer living being like himself—but both do not function as authentically traumatic encounters.

Through the prism of the Real and the imaginary, we can begin to approach the foundational procedure of animal trauma—a traumatic event gains its status as such due to its tearing (from within) of the imaginary fabric that is constitutive of animal subjectivity and accordingly structures their phenomenality. With Eslom's trauma, it is unequivocally apparent that a purely positivist neurological explanation elides proper apprehension of the kernel of subjective imaginary attachment initiating the PTSD response: As discussed, the familial identification with the mother *as mother* (along with Eslom's corresponding imaginary sense of self) prompts the traumatic character of the loss—without this element, the death would be devoid of its utterly staggering and disorienting radicality; it is the Real embedded in the event and its overbearing contact with the imaginary field that renders it truly traumatic.

The study on elephant trauma offers a similar structural effect of a puncturing of the imaginary field by a traumatic Real. As the researcher's noted, they could not fully attribute the PTSD-like symptomology to the loss of kinship based learning (transferential learning) since the loss (of family members, or others in their communal tribe) itself was traumatic—and despite those researchers relying exclusively on the positivist-neuronal understanding of trauma (because the experience and its sustained impact was indeed traumatic for the elephants, rather than its effects merely being a consequence of a lack of learned behavior) the register of the Real overtaking the imaginary supplies a more immediate explication that accounts for the phenomenology of trauma. Again, the conception of the Real and its relation to the animal imaginary tells us not what occurs in some brain region associated with certain behaviors, but instead *why something is traumatic in the first place*. While traumatic events are normally described as 'overwhelming,' a Lacanian conception of animal subjectivity delineates *what is being overwhelmed* and how this traumatizing surplus of experience is distinct from a human's trauma (an animal trauma is the Real overtaking the imaginary; a human trauma is the Real overtaking the symbolic).

If the traumatic Real's intervention in animal subjectivity relies on an imaginary bound up with its implacable social identifications and conceptions-of-self (or, at the least, an awareness of self, structured by the imaginary field), then how does continual fear-inducing stimuli, such as the audio of a natural predator for the chickadees, function as a traumatic event? In what sense is this an overtaking of the imaginary? By a certain interpretation, this confirms the commonsensical view of trauma: The sonic stimuli (conceived as a traumatic Real) overtakes (as in rendering the senses incapable of assimilating the sensory input) the imaginary field, generating an unapproachable hole that seems totally alien to the very domain of its origin (a sonic emission doubtlessly resides in the imaginary sphere within the recipient), exiling the animal (in a sense) from their own (imaginary) subjective network. Is this not precisely what one means when they cast the traumatic as an event that is 'too much' or 'overwhelming' to the subject?

We should be reminded at this juncture of the distinction between a psychical trauma and a purely physical trauma: A physical trauma is defined not in relation to a subjectivity but is rather constituted on the bodily-empirical plane—an injury is traumatic in an immediate, perceptual sense and is known through its objectivity in 'reality' as such. Simply, a train colliding with a human (or animal) body and irrevocably crushing multiple limbs is not traumatic (on the plane of physicality) merely because one's consciousness cannot contend with the notion of a train striking a body; the collision is corporeally traumatic because it literally overcomes the bounded limits of the body. As Freud articulates it, physical trauma is "the result of the protective shield having been broken through in a limited area,"[43] leading to a flood of un-pleasure. Two subjectivities—assuming the same position, placement, and speed of train—would undergo the same physical trauma if struck, but we observe that a psychical trauma operates according to a dissimilar procedure: The event being an instantiation of that which is traumatic is contingent on an explosively intrusive relation to an individual subjectivity (like fireworks for the veteran with PTSD). To refer to the research on the traumatized chickadees—the noise issuing from the audio playback speakers is not traumatic in its literal materiality (like the train colliding with the human body—since the predator is only present through auditory mimicry) but rather is traumatic *in its subjective reception.* For the chickadees, the noise is clearly traumatic because it is identical (as a recording) to the sound cast by their predators, and to another subject (such as a human subject) the noise would not be perceived as traumatic, being easily assimilated into their symbolic network. An endlessly replayed sound (for 48 hours) of a predator's call for a captive chickadee is traumatic insofar as it shatters its imaginary structure—what is 'too much' is precisely the sonic act that functions as the Real, with the imaginary unable to assimilate it. The imaginary field is unable to account for the traumatic sensory-event.

Physical and psychic trauma cannot be entirely severed into a totalizing dichotomous split. Cases such as the torture of the rats and their dreams attest that there are instances where corporeal suffering and subjective-interior trauma overlap and are concomitant. The distinction between physical trauma—like getting hit by a train—and non-objective, subjectively-felt psychic trauma, is not to render these into two distinct arenas of trauma (and to implicitly neglect the subjective trauma that arises from physical abuse and torture), but instead to assert that trauma cannot be simplified to a physiological response in the animal, and that the traumatic Real is indissoluble to objective events. The objective event—no matter how physically painful—requires a subjectivity that is unable to index, through whatever means, the encounter with inexplicably impossible suffering. The rat's physical pain is traumatic, not because of its effects on the materiality of the body, but because of its effects on the structure of the rat's subjectivity.

The contemporary discovery of animal PTSD in fields such as biology, zoology, and animal psychology affirms yet another dimension of the Real: its definitional propensity for repetition. The Real is, as noted at the start of the chapter, "that which always comes back to the same place," and the subject returns to the Real again and again, endlessly. Is this not the very constitutive characteristic of PTSD that brings recognition of its symptomology and renders it the subject of the cultural imagination? PTSD is the re-emergence of the traumatic material, again and again, into waking (and sleeping) reality—and it is precisely this fact that makes PTSD the ideal vessel for narrativization of trauma and mental illness. In Lacanian terms, within the scope of the human, PTSD is an encounter with the (initial) unbearable Real spurring the recurring re-appearance of the Real in the register of the symbolic as a conspicuous fracture in the symbolic network that language perpetually and tragically circles and fails to designate. The reiterative re-appearance of the Real is exactly what the animal experiences in instances of PTSD-like 'cluster symptoms': the negative alteration in Eslom's behavior, for instance, years after the traumatic loss of his mother and sister, is indicative of a stressor in the structural field that does not merely result in a one-time encounter but rather an unremitting re-encounter, haunting the imaginary field that structures his subjectivity. Animal PTSD, like human PTSD, is the eternal wound of consciousness that the structural field tries to treat, and its inability to cover this lesion generates an even more festering injury—a wound that (seemingly) does not close and only reproduces itself in the same spot.

The ineluctable insight is this: Animal trauma cannot be reduced to its objective dimension (unlike the physical trauma of an injury) and must be contended with as a psychic phenomenality on the individuated level of subjectivity. If animals experience trauma (which modern research unequivocally affirms), then there is a specific interiority that collapses, in some way, under an experience, and the Lacanian registers—specifically for animals, the register of the imaginary—offer a structural understanding of that experience (of trauma) and its relation to animal subjectivity. Animals experience trauma, along with its lasting effects, because their subjectivity is structured by the imaginary field—and this field, while mediating the Real, also permits its intrusion, implicitly embedded in the imaginary's very limitations as a structural site.

The Real is the *reason* an event is traumatic—whether for an animal or for a human. An encounter with an externalized act (an empirical act that occurs in the 'out-there' beyond any individuated subjectivity), always exceeds the field that structures subjectivity (whether that is an animal subjectivity constituted by the imaginary field or a human subjectivity constituted by the symbolic field) is not necessarily traumatic unless it is a Real capable of puncturing the constitutive field (the register of the symbolic or imaginary). Again, this is why a psychic trauma implicates a subjectivity that is 'overwhelmed': A non-sentient robot who is hit by a train will incur a physical 'trauma' (a sustained limp, for instance) *despite the fact they are devoid of subjectivity* because that modality of trauma is not contingent on subjectivity. However, not only does the experience of trauma indicate an underlying subjectivity that is irrevocably pierced, but it also permits us to theorize on *those very subjective structural contents which are pierced and precisely what pierces them*. An animal experiences trauma due to the internal limits of the imaginary register—which, when attempting to contend with an event that cannot be designated by the imaginary network (an event that surpasses the imaginary's limit), becomes an unassimilable Real, haunting the imaginary field and enabling the PTSD-like symptoms found in the newest research on animals. However, an animal's experience of the Real is not exhausted by trauma since the Real is not strictly a negative phenomenon—there is also a jouissance of animality.

From Trauma to Jouissance: The Real Enjoyment of Animality

Animal trauma stages an entry-point into animality and the Real—demonstrating, quite straightforwardly, that the animal Real is mediated by the imaginary register (an analogous structural feature parallel to the human's Real mediated by the symbolic)—but trauma is not the terminating point for the animal Real. For animals, like humans, the Real remains bound to subjective experience itself—particularly in its emergence as a mode of jouissance, with all of its connections to the body as a site exceeding the binding force of the imaginary and the symbolic. Bruce Fink explains that the real, in this a-traumatic sense, is a "seamless surface" that includes the body:

> The real is, for example, an infant's body 'before' it comes under the sway of the symbolic order, before it is instructed to toilet training and subjected to the ways of the world . . . the real is a sort of unrent, undifferentiated fabric, woven in such a way to be full everywhere . . . . It is a sort of smooth, seamless surface or space which applies as much to a child's body as to the whole universe.[44]

Like Lacan, Fink defines the Real as "*that which is not yet* symbolized, remains to be symbolized, or even resists symbolization."[45] Returning to the discussion in the preceding section, we recall that the Real is contextualized, by psychoanalytic theorists and Lacan himself, through the human register of the symbolic—and that is why, for Fink, the pre-linguistic state of infant-hood is taken to be a time immersed in the Real. However, one must be reminded to avoid the temptation to situate animals in the time of the infant 'before' the symbolic: The infant is not only pre-linguistic (pre-symbolic), but they are also largely pre-imaginary, meaning nothing (or, at least not much) is there to mediate between the infant and the Real. To re-cover territory that has, by this point, been utterly, painfully exhausted: This does not apply to the animal because their lack of signifier is not a developmentally incomplete stage—the absence of the symbolic is a developmental, even ontological, preclusion. Unlike the human infant, who temporarily resides in a phase of incompleteness they later conquer, an animal's lack of signifier is not a true 'lack' in the sense that there is no subjective mechanism that is 'missing' linguistic acquisition since the animal is, instead, equipped with the imaginary register to mediate and structure their reality. Recognizing that animals are not lacking creatures (who are evolutionarily or biologically stunted or in-progress) but rather are developed with their own subjective structural and topological composition eschews the proposition that animals, like the pre-linguistic infant, experience an endless expanse of Real in all its undifferentiated immediacy. If this were the case, then animals would be unable to navigate spatially or form attachments to certain objects over others—since reality (which is, for them, imputed by the register of the imaginary) would not exist and only a vast, indistinct "unrent" Real governed by instinct would exist.

The crucial insight lies in embodiment: the infant's corporeality is a site of the Real (along with the totality of existence), and even when the infant enters the symbolic domain, thereby subjecting the Real of the body into a process where "the body is progressively written or overwritten with signifiers,"[46] there nonetheless is a lingering remainder that eludes language. Like the example of sex in the prior section on trauma, we can appeal to the simple truism that events and things do not fully capitulate to language, although they can be "overwritten with signifiers." The body is a Real that exists outside of the reality aggregated for the human by language—and the same can be said of animals: their bodies, while a part of the imaginary constructions that populate their subjectivities, also exceed those constructions and present a Real that tears through the imaginary network. The animal body does not capitulate to the imaginary field, piercing the very structure of (imaginary) reality. If we remain tethered to the Real as traumatic, we cannot account for this dimension of the Real. What is this non-traumatic instantiation of the bodily Real? It is the domain of *animal jouissance.*

The dimension of the Real must occupy those reality-piercing moments, not only of the fearful-painful or traumatic, but also the pleasurable and the excessive. A traumatic incision in the mediating imaginary of animals is, clearly, an excessive, overwrought experience (an intrusion of the Real)—but what of an experience that is excessive in the opposing direction: Does the pole of pleasure not lead us to a role of jouissance in the subjective structure of animality? A mode of jouissance outside of the networks of signifier and the imaginary aligns perfectly with what Jacques-Alain Miller calls *impossible jouissance* "which means real jouissance," a jouissance that is "attributed to the Real."[47] Impossible jouissance is the facticity of corporeality that forever exceeds the other registers that impotently attempt to contain it. To provide a fairly straightforward illustration of jouissance for humans, consider the libido and the fundamental Lacanian demarcation between pleasure and jouissance:

> We see clearly here the opposition between libido transcribed as desire, where it appears between the signifiers, and libido as *das Ding*, where it appears beyond signifier and signified.[48]

Jouissance is precisely that modality of libido that "appears beyond" the symbolic network, while traditional libido remains "transcribed as desire," and is submitted to the signifier and the Law which subtends it. Jouissance is libido that has not been submitted to Law—a desire that cannot be contained by the symbolic field; it cannot be subdued by symbolization. For humans, a loss of the most radical and immediate degree of jouissance is a pre-condition for civilization. Human civilization is predicated on relinquishing the libidinal desire that is unbounded by Law; 'anti-social,' non-symbolizable jouissance must be ceded so that 'pro-social,' symbolizable desire can be formed.

Abandoning excessive libidinal desire in the name of the foundation of human civilization is a basic tenet of Freudian psychoanalysis, certainly antecedent to Lacanian psychoanalysis, and one of Freud's famous universalized 'myths' (the patricide of the primal horde's Father) centers on the notion of surrendering excessive enjoyment in exchange for a pro-social pleasure principle. In *Civilization and Its Discontents*, Freud introduces this patricide, insisting that it is *the* originating event of all civilizations. Freud observes that Darwin's famous primal horde must have been controlled by a "violent and jealous father who keeps all the females for himself and drives away his sons as they grow up."[49] Eventually, through some enigmatic "cultural advance," the sons "who had been driven out came together, killed and devoured their father and so made an end of the patriarchal horde," and this "criminal deed" becomes "the beginning of so many things—of social organization, of moral restrictions and of religion."[50] Lacan affirms the centrality of the killing of the primordial father in Freud's thought, writing in *Écrits* that he perceived it to be "the inaugural drama of humanity."[51]

Crucially, Freud notes that the patricide was the impetus for the creation of Law based on a familial social organization that privileged the majority rather than the minority:

> Though the brothers had banded together in order to overcome their father, they were all one another's rivals in regard to the women. Each of them would have wished, like his father, to have all the women to himself. The new organization would have collapsed in a struggle of all against all, for none of them was of such overmastering strength as to be able to take on his father's part with success. Thus the brothers had no alternative, if they were to live together, but—not, perhaps, until they had passed through many dangerous crises—to institute the law against incest, by which they all alike renounced the women whom they desired and who had been their chief motive for despatching their father. In this way they rescued the organization which had made them strong.[52]

To sustain living together post-patricide, the brothers must "institute" the injunction against incest, thereby permitting more harmonious relations, with certain women being rendered beyond 'legal' sexual access—meaning prohibited by a collective force surpassing any one brother. Do we not see in Freud's mythic theory the exact same hydraulic mechanism at play between jouissance and libido? Jouissance is brought to an end by a Law (enacted through the symbolic—signified and conceptualized) that limits enjoyment to a socially sanctioned desire.

Here, we encounter the Lacanian notion of castration in the register of the Real: Earlier (in Chapter 1), we found that castration was, for Lacan, the severance between the subject and unmediated experience (the Real) brought about by the unrelenting mediation of language (generating symbolic reality), and we find here the principle (of language resulting in an estrangement from the Real) applied to the social dimension and jouissance—to enter into civilization, the subject is castrated by Law. And what, exactly, is excised by this form of implicit socialization-castration? It is precisely the excessive, undomesticated jouissance that refuses to submit to language and its Law. André Green concisely states that civilization is based on a "renunciation" which "never finds compensation equal to the sacrifices to which it must consent."[53] We give up the endless expanse of jouissance and are given in return civilized enjoyment. Lacan's paradigm of castration and jouissance is a signifier-centric recapitulation of the Freudian primordial patricide understood through the Symbolic and Law, with jouissance being the pre-civilized excessive enjoyment of the primal father, and castration being the condition all subsequent subjects must submit to in order to remain bound by the ties of fraternalization (on whatever plane it appears—either locally and concrete, or nationally and diffuse). Lacan states this quite clearly in *Écrits*, writing that:

> We must keep in mind that jouissance is prohibited to whoever speaks, as such—or, put differently, it can only be said between the lines by whoever is a subject of the Law, since the Law is founded on that very prohibition.[54]

Lacan writes, in a very direct and lucid manner, that jouissance is outside the symbolic bounds of the speaking being (the human)—and that the Law (constitutive of human civilization and any degree of social cohesion) is "founded" on expelling jouissance. Yet, Lacan goes further, reminding us that, "it is not the Law itself that bars the subject's access to jouissance . . . . For it is pleasure that sets limits to jouissance, pleasure as what binds incoherent life together."[55] Lacan returns here to the foundational opposition between pleasure and jouissance: pleasure limits one's access to jouissance and acts as its boundary. Everything outside of pleasure, in the register of enjoyment, is the domain of jouissance.

Jouissance, as an enjoyment that exceeds pleasure, has two interrelated procedures. In one sense, jouissance is that which is outside the Law that regulates desire (it is the primal father exiling his sons and keeping all the women for himself—an unsustainable modality of enjoyment that precludes and supersedes social intersubjectivity). For the sake of fraternalization and civilization, this form of jouissance must be given up (like the brothers, who after the death of the father, limit their incestuous jouissance in the name of a reality principle of communally regulated libido)—and, of course, this is initiated through language: As the subject enters language, the Law of regulation (i.e., castration) is transmitted. This is why, for Lacan, the entrance into the symbolic order is analogous to a second birth: "we are, as it were, born a second time, in leaving behind the state which is rightly known as the *infans* sate, for it is without speech."[56] The significance of this 'second birth' is not merely speech's import as a means of conceptual intersubjective exchange—it is also what that exchange heralds for the subject, namely the incorporation of a Law, subsequently determining (in a not insubstantial manner) their being. Consider the child who must cease the enjoyment associated with freely relieving themselves in their diaper, with a parent directing them to instead use 'the potty'—and the entire scene is punctuated by the flow of signifiers such as, *Good job!* and *Let's try again*—is their otherwise unregulated enjoyment not now regulated by a Law of excrement (that comes with its own, limited, pleasure of shit-evacuation)?

In the second sense (which is, undoubtedly, attached to the first), jouissance is a form of enjoyment that *literally* exceeds pleasure and the pleasure principle. Lacan defines the pleasure principle as a law that

> fixes the level of a certain quantity of excitation which cannot be exceeded without going beyond the limit of the *Lust/Unlust* polarity—pleasure and unpleasure are the only two forms through which that same and single mode of regulation we call the pleasure principle expresses itself.[57]

Simply, the pleasure principle is predicated on aversion to un-pleasure (pain, deprivation, etc.) and the concurrent movement towards that which is pleasurable—and once one surpasses "a certain quantity of excitation," they find themselves either in a state of displeasure, or a state of jouissance (which may not always be incompatible). Crucially, the pleasure principle's horizon, its hold on subjectivity, is complicated by the reality principle. Freud introduced the reality principle to designate the human psychic mediation of the pleasure principle: The reality principle takes into account not only pleasure or unpleasure (the lust/unlust binary), but also the social implications and ramifications which arise from a given act. Freud states in his introductory lectures that the reality principle "at bottom seeks to obtain pleasure, but pleasure which is assured through taking account of reality, even though it is pleasure postponed and diminished."[58] Reality imposes restraints on one's search for pleasure—limiting the avenues of pleasure that one will pursue.

It should be apparent how the reality principle is concurrently distinct, yet related, to the symbolic Law: The reality principle forms the bounds of pleasure—it is not necessarily the prohibitions themselves, but rather the ways a social reality places a parameter around pleasure, functionally warning the subject that exceeding the socially-generated parameter may result in a reduction of pleasure. Something analogous to: *If I engage in X, my long-term pleasure will ultimately undergo a diminution.* While the function of the reality principle overlaps with the Law, they are not strictly collapsible into each other—since both consist of semi-distinct operations. The reality principle, along with the pleasure principle, distills the tension of the subject at the boundary of pleasure. We can detect, then, three economies of pleasure (albeit we must observe an interdependence between them for the human subject): The raw pleasure principle; the pleasure principle overlaid with the reality principle; and the symbolic Law. Jouissance is the enjoyment (transcending the limit of pleasure) that drastically overrides all three of these structural libidinal economies of satisfaction.

In this sense, jouissance is an enjoyment-beyond-pleasure—a mode of enjoyment that is 'too much' for the subject, straddling the very precipice that demarcates the division of pleasure and pain. Lacan emphasizes the excessive force of jouissance in his seminar *The Four Fundamental Concepts*, writing that "there is a *jouissance* beyond the pleasure principle."[59] Lacan also states clearly that, "unquestionably, there is jouissance at the level which pain begins to appear, and we know that it is only at this level of pain that a whole dimension of the organism, which would otherwise remain veiled, can be experienced."[60] Without even considering the position of Law, or the reality principle, jouissance is enjoyment exceeding pleasure in its raw state. T.R. Johnson refers to this excessive enjoyment-beyond-pleasure as "those pleasures that share in the death drive—the ecstasy of the suicide bomber."[61] Implicit in jouissance is painful—even lethal—non-pleasures.

But there arises a reasonable objection: How can there be a modality of enjoyment that overrides the principle of pleasure itself? In a scene from the children's movie, *Matilda*,[62] about a maltreated orphan, the limits of pleasure are perfectly articulated. A young boy, Bruce, is accused of stealing a piece of cake by the hyper-punitive, tyrannical para-military principle, Miss Trunchbull, and is then (counterintuitively) reprimanded by being made to eat a large slice of chocolate cake in front of the entire assembled school in the auditorium—and once he apprehensively yields, Bruce derives clear gastronomic pleasure from the cake; he enjoys it in the conventional sense. Once Bruce finishes the slice, he is presented with an enormous chocolate cake, Miss Trunchbull informing him that he must finish the entire cake, thereby delivering a torturous twist on the standard punishment of deprivation, instead moving onto the opposing axis of excess. Suddenly, the desired object that generated pleasure (the slice of cake) becomes an excessive site that surpasses pleasure into punishment engendered by the ostensibly insurmountable challenge (a mode of psychic pain). After initially nearing failure, almost unable to finish the cake, he is eventually supported by the spectating students, who begin chanting his name—and finally finishes the cake to the applause of his classmates, licking the now-empty tray of cake clean.

Bruce's triumph, and eventual enjoyment, of the deployment of excess for punitive means (the huge cake, used to render the object of his desire as totally undesirable), is a perfect paradigm for apprehending jouissance: Finishing the cake defied both the Law and the inherent limits of the pleasure principle, bringing him a mode of enjoyment that goes *beyond* these economies. When Bruce finishes the first slice of cake, Miss Trunchbull mockingly offers him more—to which he says no, that he is full and has had enough. This gesture is, of course, indicative of pleasure's standard limit of satisfaction: He had eaten the slice and was satisfied. In a similar manner, by converting a punishment into a victorious act, he contravened the Law and experienced what could be called the rebel's jouissance that defies Law. One should note, though, that this superimposition of excessive punishment onto the former site of pleasure is not a form of conventional pleasure—since the boy clearly does not derive enjoyment from the act itself but rather its violative crossing of the threshold of Law and pleasure. Despite the 'too-muchness' inherent in the act of eating the entire chocolate cake, the boy achieves an enjoyment that can be assigned a status as jouissance proper.

As we see in the emblematic scene from *Matilda*, and as Lacan reminds us, it is not only 'Law' that limits jouissance—it is also pleasure itself. We can accordingly localize jouissance in two poles of *beyond*: 'Beyond' the Law that regulates the conditions of individuated desire, and 'beyond' the pleasure principle that organizes the libidinal economy (with its governing agency of auto-moderating homeostasis, recoiling from a non-pleasurable immoderation oriented towards a pleasurable sensation that presents itself as unlimited). The excessiveness of jouissance, overriding both poles of Law and pleasure, situates it as an experience squarely in the domain of the Real. The pleasure principle and the Law are both situated in the spheres of the imaginary and the symbolic—and accordingly the 'beyond' of these spheres (which jouissance brings to the subject) is that of the Real.

Recognition of jouissance as an experience in the Real permits the introduction of an animal jouissance: Do animals not, like humans, have a pleasure principle that organizes their libidinal economies? What would it mean for this principle to be violated in the name of further enjoyment—an enjoyment-beyond-pleasure? We can begin by stating this: Similar to how the Real in the experience of trauma in animals is an event that supersedes the imaginary register—eluding its direct-representational grasp—the Real in the experience of jouissance overcomes the mediator of reality and presents an absolute disjuncture from everyday reality (the Real pierces reality in a non-traumatic directionality). However, a few things must be qualified to tidy up the discourse before we proceed in this direction of animal subjectivity and jouissance in the register of the Real.

First, it should be clear that the jouissance of animals is not contingent at all on a symbolic Law that situates their behavior in the realm of moral values: There is not, for the animal, an equivalent to the postulated originary patricide and subsequent moral development (a communal-collective agreement to limit their range of behavior) that Freud assigns to humanity. Animal behavior is, instead, unfettered by a symbolic Law—although, as we have seen, they are not entirely outside the imaginary bounds of a lesser iteration of guilt and punishment. The fact that animals are not submitted to a symbolic Law does not mean, of course, that they do not participate in social organizations that prohibit behaviors or promote (or even demand) other behaviors. An ant participates in a social organization of the collective colony that includes submission to an order and certain 'rules'—albeit these rules should not necessarily be classified as Laws in the Lacanian or more general psychoanalytic sense. Ants, for instance, engage in different tasks according to the needs of the nest, and though this is done independently of any direct delegation (ants do not inform another ant of what they must do—they are not directed to a new task in a hierarchical manner), the ants do adhere to signs (of other ants' behavior) that coordinate their innate task-related behavior.

Scholars studying the normative behavior of ants write that "ethological research points to the existence of rules that coordinate the temporal subdivision of activities in order to change work allocation according to the changing needs of the colony."[63] Specifically, they explain that ants discern if a task should be continued or abandoned based on the behavior of other ants:

> Ants are thus capable of making clear behavioral changes by switching from one activity to another, according to a "rule" made possible by the cognitive ability to perceive the number of a certain kind of individuals encountered in certain situations.[64]

It is essential to invoke here a distinction between an externally imposed normative rule (and a pre-installed instinct guiding behavior) from symbolic Law as such: A symbolic Law comes with a secondary plane of prohibitions radically exceeding the flattened sign. First, because a symbolic Law relies on language (the signifier) for its transmission, and secondly because Law involves embeddedness in the human conscious mechanism that results in repression and ultimately the content of the unconscious. The entire classical Freudian psychoanalytical framework is derived from this conception of Law. Consequently, other animals' social organizations, such as ants or even those with clearer norms such as apes, do not operate according to a symbolic Law as human civilizations do.

Animals would not find enjoyment-beyond-pleasure in the breaking of Law because they do not obey that symbolic Law in the first place—animals do not participate in what Lacan calls *transgressive jouissance*. To again reference an earlier example: The dog that chews on the shoe—despite the punishment that ensues from engaging in a prohibited act—does not experience an enjoyment that exceeds the role of pleasure (jouissance) because there is not a symbolic Law that is transgressed: the dog derives the exact same enjoyment from chewing on a non-prohibited shoe as a prohibited one (aside from some actual differential between the shoes that would augment pleasure). Yet (the objection goes) how can we know what the dog subjectively experiences when they engage in prohibited acts? Here, we must refer again to the distinction between pre-super-egoic guilt and super-egoic guilt proper (from Chapter 1): The guilt that the dog experiences is immanent to the external punishment, along with an imaginary identification (as worthy of love—as a 'good dog'); a super-egoic guilt (a Law dispensed from the register of the symbolic) relies on an internally installed sense of guilt that pervades consciousness and can be detached from the external action, instead inhabiting the phantasies and thoughts of the subject. Guilt exists on the plane of thought for the human (sanctioned by the superego); for animals, it exists in the external world of actions and punishments. Consequently, the notion of animal jouissance resides in the second boundary that jouissance crosses, namely, the boundary of pleasure itself.

Where does the excessive power of jouissance appear in animal experience? In a basic and elementary way, we can turn to an example similar to the chocolate cake scene from *Matilda*: It is clear that animals will cross the threshold of pleasure to reach *supra-enjoyment* (a term I use to designate a fixture of jouissance as an enjoyment that exceeds the pleasure principle). A common scene from a domesticated pet illustrates the operation of enjoyment-beyond-pleasure for animals—when an animal-pet, for instance a hamster, dog, or fish, is provided with a hyper-abundance of food, rather than limiting themself to the limit of pleasure-satisfaction, they will exceed this pleasure into a post-pleasure enjoyment (jouissance). In short, when provided with food, certain animals will not cease eating until they are physically unable to do so, beyond the point of satiation.

The conditions for animal obesity only emerge through a conjunction of a superabundance of resources, high-fat foods, and low-activity levels, meaning animal obesity only arrives through human intervention in environmental processes. Comparative Psychologists Daniel C. Marston and Terry L. Maple explain: "Obesity is not common throughout the animal world . . . domesticated animals are the only other animal population to have obesity to any noteworthy degree."[65] Alexander J. German notes that "obesity . . . is the most common nutritional disorder in companion animals"[66] and that obesity, specifically in cats (although this can presumably be applied to other domesticated animals as well), can be caused by "failure to develop control of satiety."[67] Marston and Maple also link overeating to an inability for self-control over satiation—blaming this "failure" on addiction. They reference studies in which animals exhibited "neurochemical changes associated with addiction" and rats "who had continuous access to fatty foods would binge on those foods."[68] Both these examples, *Matilda* and the pet who eats-towards-obesity, appeal to a modality of hunger that transcends need, satisfaction, and pleasure: They are demonstrative of the jouissance of obesity.

Does obesity not present us with this peculiar hunger-beyond-hunger which undermines—or patently subverts—the function of hunger as a means to sustaining life? The pet's hunger, as an instinct, goes against the very evolutionary utility it holds when the domesticated animal eats until they reach—or even surpass—the precipice of pleasure (consider the accompanying health issues that emerge from obesity). Further, should we not ascertain that the pet derives some enjoyment, that exceeds conventional pleasure, in what is ultimately an eating-towards-death? If not enjoyment (in terms of jouissance), what mechanism compels the animal to eat past the edge of pleasure? One could appeal, here, to the diffuse notion of 'instinct' (that the instinct to eat putatively impels the animal towards obesity when food is hyper-abundantly present)—yet is instinct not bounded, most of all, to the guiding biological principle of self-preservation; and accordingly, how would a mechanism operating towards the conservation of life use that very instinct in a movement towards a diametrically opposed purpose? We should recognize, at this juncture, a shared *jouissance* between animality and humanity: A jouissance that plows past the pleasure principle.

As I have been vigilant in observing throughout this section, the structures of animal and human pleasure are certainly distinct: Human pleasure is structured by the symbolic and animal pleasure is structured by the imaginary. One could object here and answer: *yes, pleasure may be structured—but its* limit *is surely biological.* We arrive here at a nearly unequivocal concession to biology—pleasure's limits are certainly constrained by a biological reality that determines its boundaries. If need is determined by biological mechanisms, then so is the boundary of when pleasure slips into a non-pleasure or anti-pleasure. However, this does not functionally negate the insight into pleasure as operating in a particular subjective topological register: Consider the function of language in human pleasure, for instance. Does the qualifier (issued from the site of speech) of 'ice-cold drink,' dispatched by an advertisement (such as a Coca-Cola advertisement played before a movie), not enhance the pleasure one obtains from drinking it? Further, what about the desires that are derived from the Other, determinative of human desire? As Lacan writes, "desire is the desire of the Other,"[69] and the transmission from the Other (understood as the "locus of speech") to the subject occurs, clearly, through language and the symbolic field. Even sexual desires and their supposedly instinctual nature are mediated through the symbolic universe: The breast (or the phallus) is not merely an inert object that one is drawn to (is desired) only out of biological 'hardwiring'—these objects of desire are bound up in the signifiers that overlay them, both orienting and designating human pleasure. Without the symbolic, human desire would be indistinguishable from animal intercourse; reproductive copulatory activity would be the definitive end of all human sexual relations. Fetish and obsessions would not exist.

Animal pleasure, while not operating on the plane of the symbolic through human language, is not totally unmediated either. The role of the imaginary network, in terms of a sensory domain, is clear in animal's relation to food: A cat detects the sound wet can of food opening, setting off a desperate reaction; a treat bag, making a particular sound, will elicit a greater response than the ordinary bag of food (these are obvious insights that animal pleasure is bound up with sensory perceptions). More deeply embedded in the role of conventional animal pleasure is the position of imaginary identifications in the process of sexual relations. The most famed, and ostentatious example is the (male) peacock, displaying flamboyant colors and designs to signal a certain degree of health or vigor to the (female) peahen. As is well-known (albeit initially contested), Charles Darwin's assertion in *Sexual Selection and the Descent of Man*[70] is that peahens select the peacocks with the most flamboyant design, leading to a propagation of the genetic mutation that results in the noted trains. Marion Petrie, Tim Halliday, and Carolyn Sanders, the first researchers to empirically confirm Darwin's claim on peacocks and sexual selection in 1991, write in their paper:

> Our results show that there is non-random mating in peafowl, that a large part of the variance in mating success can be attributed to variance in train morphology and that females choose to mate with those males that have the most elaborate trains of those sampled.[71]

As the study shows, peahens are drawn to peacocks with the most elaborate, colorful designs on their plumage—and this shows an imaginary representational identification: The selection of a mate (i.e., animal attraction) occurs on the plane of the scopic. Through the visual landscape, the entire arena of sexual relations and reproductive mating erupts. Or, even, to reference again Lacan's pigeons: The developmental moment of sexual maturation is initiated by a species-level identification occurring in the visual sphere.

The imaginary register's role in animal pleasure, like the symbolic's place in human pleasure, is undeniable; the imaginary is fundamentally constitutive of animal pleasure. Here, then, one must ask: How does jouissance manage to overcome the imaginary network in the first place? One could attempt to situate animal jouissance in a mere lack of discernment—that animals cannot recognize the limits of pleasure as a human does and so they inadvertently surpass that limit—not due to the pursuit of an enjoyment-beyond-pleasure—but instead a failure to discriminate the boundary of pleasure and pain; while it is certainly true that they cannot reflect on this limit, the limit of pleasure is *sensed* in the exact way a human limit of pleasure is sensed as an intuitive, sensory biological boundary. Logically, then, a jouissance of animality surpasses the biological boundary of pleasure that is designated by the imaginary field. By an intervention from the Real, which emerges from the very convergence of the biological sphere and the imaginary field, the jouissance of animality is made possible. This psychoanalytic formula explains the propensity for animal enjoyment to violate the pleasure principle: Not only do animals experience jouissance, *but they are also even more prone to its disastrous results.* But why is there more direct access to a deadly form of jouissance-beyond-pleasure for animals? For instance, the domesticated animal that eats itself to death-through-obesity—plainly violating the reality principle and pleasure principle. Reference to human domestication of animals and the attendant access to an overabundance of resources does not suffice to explain the jouissance of animals—the fact of animals encountering an overabundance and subsequently over-indulging does not answer *why* their enjoyment does not cease at the limit of pleasure. Instead, we must appeal to a process that has no bearing on animal subjectivity (this lack-of-lack permits a liquid state of jouissance in animality): Castration and the phallic symbol.

Humans, as delineated earlier, are castrated and severed from jouissance; animals are, crucially, the very opposite of castrated: They instead, and have a more direct access to jouissance—an animal jouissance. Humans are castrated, generally (to say nothing of sexual relations or Oedipal triangles), in two interrelated ways: They are castrated by the symbolic (the signifier mediating experientiality) and by the Law imposed on the plane of sociality (a communal 'social contract' that limits one's range of pleasure, thus establishing taboos). Lacan outlines that humans "by their nature as fully developed beings, speaking beings, are castrated."[72] Precisely here is where the phallus is introduced as a forever-unobtainable symbolic object of non-castrated jouissance: The phallus is jouissance's signifier as that which is lacked. As Lacan says, quite simply, "the phallus is a signifier."[73] Crucially, the 'true' phallus (and its concomitant jouissance) can never be secured—it is irrecoverable, forever lost as one enters into sociality and the symbolic universe. Lacan reminds us, "man cannot aim at being whole . . . once the play of displacement and condensation to which he is destined in the exercise of his functions marks his relation, as a subject, to the signifier,"[74] and the phallic signifier symbolically marks this un-wholeness: "the phallus serves the function of signifying the lack of being that is wrought in the subject by his relation to the signifier."[75] Human lack, our "deprivation or not-being" is "symbolized by the phallus."[76]

The phallus, in its 'true dimension' as a non-symbolic access to fullness and jouissance beyond the reality and pleasure principle, cannot be obtained because "language and the law of language take it away from him."[77] Even to speak of the phallus in this way, as some lost-object, is a fantasy: There was no pure phallic 'before' language—the concept of a return is a falsely retroactive re-construction only available in its phantasmic dimension after the entrance into the symbolic universe. Situating animals in relation to the phallus is tricky for precisely this reason. Animals are not castrated, yet they do not have a phallic signifier (because they do not have access to the signifier *and* because their un-castrated state leaves them without need for this symbolic designation).

Animals being uncastrated is where we find the immediacy in animality that humans are frequently jealous of; they experience a modality of enjoyment that humans cannot, due to animals not being submitted to the castrating function of human sociality and the symbolic. Walt Whitman, in his poem "Song of Myself," expresses a post-romantic reflection on animality that exhibits a longing for their uncastrated nature:

> I think I could turn, and live with animals, they are so placid and self-contained/I stand and look at them long and long./They do not sweat and whine about their condition,/They do not lie awake in the dark and weep for their sins.[78]

Whitman deploys the poetic dimension to articulate a truth on animality that aligns with our comments on philosophy and psychoanalytic theory. Take the final line, that animals do not "lie awake in the dark and weep for their sins"—is this not an exact articulation of a certain enviousness on the side of humanity of the fact that animals are not submitted to Law and its attendant, overbearing superegoic guilt? Animals are not burdened by an internally installed superego nor the external social Law that initiates the superego's installation. Further, what do we make of animals being described as "self-contained"? Whitman is opposing the "self-contained" animal to the human who is evidently not-self-contained—and we see here a perfect analogy to the non-castrated (i.e. whole, or "self-contained") animal and the castrated (i.e. un-whole, or not-self-contained) human. The human is lacking something which they must symbolically designate at an irretrievable distance (the phallus), while the animal has no use for this symbol (nor the linguistic means to index it).

Lacan, critiquing the notion of a human aspiration for totality (as a state without lack), writes, "it is impossible for human beings to accede to an experience of totality, because they are divided and ripped apart, no analysis being able to restore totality."[79] In different terms, Lacan comes to the same conclusion as Whitman: That humans do not have access to a totality of experience (of being self-contained) due to language and the concomitant function of Law. In Lacanian phallic terms, animals are un-castrated (without any need for the phallus-as-signifier), while humans are castrated (with a reliance on the phallus-as-signifier). The human encounter with animal being is a distinct encounter with an irreconcilable modality of lack: Human's lack (they are castrated, relying on the symbolic to mediate experience), but animals *lack* lack; in a sense, animals have a lack-of-lack that is simultaneously subjected to the envy of humanity, and in a gesture that does not negate that envy, stimulates the perspective of animals as inferior beings, in their "self-contained" fullness and Law-less-ness. However, as it will be clear to the reader at this point, animals do not actually participate in a totality of experience in all its unmediated fullness since the imaginary register intervenes at various points—in different degrees, according to the animal-species—and demarcates scenes and sites of being.

To return to the original question posed on animals and the limit of pleasure: The limitless, uncastrated state of animality (in terms of Law) permits a transcendence of the pleasure principle—and this violative transcendence can only be described as a jouissance that reaches towards the Real. While the excess of animality may appear, at first glance, as a commonsensical, already-accepted truism (the basic insight that animals lack a degree of self-regulation in their behaviors when compared to humans), we should be emphatic about the radicality of this fact: There appears to be two mutually exclusive facts of animal existence at play—animals are both closely bounded to instincts, which are entangled with and informed by the pleasure principle that, as Lacan describes, possesses "a mode of operation which is precisely to avoid excess, too much pleasure,"[80] but animals also contravene the basic operation at play in this principle by foregoing the limit of pleasure. Accordingly, one cannot strictly reduce the animal's auto-abiding instinct as a transgression of the reality principle, or to its incompatibility with a 'social contract'—animal jouissance also undermines the very nature of self-preservation that the instincts seek to serve.

To evoke a final, likely familiar, example of animal jouissance: Is the experience of a female animal in a phase of sexual receptivity (and a male animal's response to that sexual receptivity) not indicative of an enjoyment that exceeds the bounds of sexual pleasure? During periods of sexual receptivity, occurring as part of a female animal's estrous cycle, animals—such as a domesticated cat or dog—there are points that clearly go beyond conventional pleasure, even entering the realm of a painful pursuit of a mate. The most obvious counter-contention is that this is not a form of jouissance at all—*the estrous cycle is nothing more than a particular hormonal configuration determined on the level of species which the individual animal involuntarily participates in through no subjective activity of themself.*

We find here that sexual receptivity is, in 'common sense,' taken to be an instinctual response to a physiological-hormonal alteration—and this is certainly accurate, but what Lacanian psychoanalysis contributes is the recognition that the effect of this instinctual change is an overpowering of the imaginary field and the parameter of pleasure designated by the 'raw' pleasure principle. Is this procedure not precisely the Real of the instinct striking at the imaginary network that structures animal pleasure along with the biological constraints that present the limits of that pleasure? For the animal, the hormonal influx is experienced as an event of the Real overtaking the imaginary—when compared to trauma, we could say that trauma (as Real) is the overwhelming encounter with an external activity that subsumes the capacity for imaginary representation and integration, while a Real such as the estrous cycle is the overwhelming encounter with an internal activity (the deployment of hormones and other physiological changes). The former (trauma) is experienced entirely in the negative (it is devoid of any enjoyment); the latter comes with a jouissance that propels its activation in the animal subject (it comes with an enjoyment-beyond-pleasure).

The estrous cycle of a female dog, for instance, consists of symptoms of restlessness and discomfort: The dog will have physical symptoms, along with behavioral effects, such as excessive licking, hyper-activity, and putting themselves in the mounting position. Many of these are signs of a certain unpleasure—a movement away from the coveted pleasurable equilibrium that any organism desires—we must recognize, though, that the symptoms of the estrous cycle are undeniably bound up with sexuality, and hence a modality of enjoyment-beyond. Does the tension of the estrous cycle not present us with the most exemplary example of an animal jouissance? An activity that, while auto-biological, involuntary, and hormonal, situates the animal in a position beyond the pleasure principle—and that we can only assume does this through an operation that can only be defined as an instantiation of the Real (insofar as it exceeds—meaning remains unassimilable to—the animal's subjective structure of the imaginary).

For some skeptical readers, there will certainly be an implicit resistance to the notion of a jouissance of animality in the sexual field—and it is certainly the case that Lacan never dedicated a complete disquisition to delineate animal jouissance. However, Lacan himself, in a four-page digression in Seminar VII, *Transference*, explicitly states that even "insects" have access to a "sexual jouissance."[81] When discussing the well-known female Praying Mantis activity of decapitating the male's head following intercourse, Lacan writes the following:

> To subjectivize the praying mantis in this case is to make an assumption which is not excessive—that it has sexual jouissance . . . . The praying mantis is perhaps, as Descartes would not have hesitated to say, a pure and simple machine, in the sense that machines take on in his terminology, which presupposes the elimination of all subjectivity. But we ourselves have no need to remain at the stage of minimalist positions. We can grant her this jouissance . . . we must imagine here that this jouissance is correlated with the decapitation of the partner that the praying mantis is supposed to know to some degree as such.[82]

Lacan, of course, is careful to distinguish between the sexual jouissance of the female praying mantis and the human, insofar as, in human jouissance, it is a fantasy propped up by the signifier—the human's jouissance, that passes pleasure's limit into extreme, even lethal, displeasure, is pre-inscribed in the symbolic. Instead, as I've claimed, Lacan situates animal sexual jouissance in the imaginary register. In the case of the praying mantis, he writes, "[i]t is clear that an image of the imaginary other as such is present in this phenomenon."[83] Later, he finally declares that the decapitating activity of the female praying mantis is indicative of jouissance because it demonstrates the "excess" of the sexual act, a "devouring surplus" that exemplifies the "paradoxical nature of instinct"[84] in animals. Instinct is not a simple propelling force of pure, progressive machination—it goes with its own paradoxes, like the paradox of jouissance, a lethal activity with copulatory activity.

In his discussion of the praying mantis, Lacan also forecloses the question of transgressive jouissance in animality. Despite the scene of the praying mantis' deadly act appearing to us as "jouissance at the other's expense" that accordingly confers it a "moral meaning," it is "only too plain to see that we are the ones who supply this moral meaning."[85] For Lacan, there is no moral (or immoral) quality to nature's preference of "jouissance to the other."[86] This is, again, why the animal cannot experience transgressive jouissance: There is no moral dimension to their acts due to the lack of symbolic Law.

Animal jouissance exhibits, like animal trauma, the presence of a Real that collides with animal subjectivity. What, then, is the point of formulating the phenomenology of animals in this way? Are we not merely taking common examples of animal behavior and superimposing a Lacanian framework on what would otherwise be a neurological, ethological, or biological explanation? No—because consolidating animal experience—and subjectivity—through the terminology of psychoanalysis offers a more intimate view of the texture of animal interiority. A psychoanalytic view of animals and their relation to the Real does not reductively capitulate to the principle of Morgan's canon—frequently deployed to simplify all accounts of animality to their simplest interpretation (meaning arbitrarily selecting the answer affording animals the least subjective space). The principle—later called a 'canon'—was delineated by the ethologist and psychologist Lloyd Morgan and is essential to many fields dealing with animality. In the refined, second version, the principle is: "In no case is an animal activity to be interpreted in terms of higher psychological processes, if it can be fairly interpreted in terms of processes which stand lower in the scale of psychological evolution and development."[87] Simply, if it is possible (and 'reasonable'), the 'activity' of animals should always be understood as (and the animal attributed with) the lowest cognitive level.

While Morgan's canon, of course, can be advantageously used to defy anthropomorphism, one should be reluctant to predicate all insights on this principle once we realize that it can be derived from a preference for the simple over the complex not due to the merits of the simpler argument, but rather due to the presupposed merits of simplicity itself (an assertion unacceptable when applied to the human). Simply, the simplest explanation is not—as is confirmed by most other disciplines—the correct explanation. In the case of animals, the simplest response would leave nothing to be said of animal interiority: animal subjectivity would be left as an uninscribed blank space—and psychoanalysis reminds us that it is not because this space is truly blank that nothing is said about it.

Notes

1 Jacques Lacan, *Écrits*, trans. Bruce Fink (New York: W. W. Norton & Company, 2006), 466.
2 Russell Grigg, "Signifiers in the Real: From Schreber to the Wolf Man," *Psychoanalysis Lacan* 4 (2020): 1.
3 Grigg, "Signifiers in the Real," 2.
4 Grigg, "Signifiers in the Real," 1. Italics in original.
5 Lacan, *Écrits*, 478.
6 Sigmund Freud, *Beyond the Pleasure Principle*, trans. James Strachey (New York: W. W. Norton & Company, 1961), 23.
7 Lacan, *Écrits*, 324.
8 Jacques Lacan, *The Four Fundamental Concepts of Psycho-Analysis: The Seminar of Jacques Lacan, Book XI*, ed. Jacques-Alain Miller, trans. Alan Sheridan (New York: W. W. Norton & Company, 1981), 167.
9 Lacan, *Four Fundamental Concepts*, 49.
10 Lacan, *Écrits*, 324.
11 Lacan, *Four Fundamental Concepts*, 49.
12 Slavoj Žižek, *For They Know Not What They Do: Enjoyment as a Political Factor* (London: Verso, 1991), 112.
13 Žižek, *For They Know Not What They Do*, 112.
14 Jim Sheridan, dir., *Brothers* (Lionsgate, 2009).
15 Žižek, *For They Know Not What They Do*, 183.
16 Hope R. Ferdowsian, Debra L. Durham, Charles Kimwele, Godelieve Kranendonk, Emily Otali, Timothy Akugizibwe, J. B. Mulcahy, Lilly Ajarova, and Cassie Meré Johnson, "Signs of Mood and Anxiety Disorders in Chimpanzees," *PLoS One* 6, no. 6 (2011): e19855, 2.
17 Ferdowsian et al., "Signs of Mood and Anxiety Disorders in Chimpanzees," e19855, 3.
18 Ferdowsian et al., "Signs of Mood and Anxiety Disorders in Chimpanzees," e19855, 9.

19 Ferdowsian et al., "Signs of Mood and Anxiety Disorders in Chimpanzees," e19855, 2.
20 Ferdowsian et al., "Signs of Mood and Anxiety Disorders in Chimpanzees," e19855, 7.
21 Ferdowsian et al., "Signs of Mood and Anxiety Disorders in Chimpanzees," e19855, 7.
22 Ferdowsian et al., "Signs of Mood and Anxiety Disorders in Chimpanzees," e19855, 7.
23 Ferdowsian et al., "Signs of Mood and Anxiety Disorders in Chimpanzees," e19855, 8.
24 Ferdowsian et al., "Signs of Mood and Anxiety Disorders in Chimpanzees," e19855, 9.
25 John Bowlby, *Attachment*, vol. 1 of *Attachment and Loss* (New York: Basic Books, 1969), 190.
26 Bowlby, *Attachment*, 191.
27 Lacan, *Écrits*, 76.
28 David M. Peña-Guzmán, *When Animals Dream: The Hidden World of Animal Consciousness* (Princeton, NJ: Princeton University Press, 2022), 94.
29 Peña-Guzmán, *When Animals Dream*, 95.
30 Peña-Guzmán, *When Animals Dream*, 97.
31 Peña-Guzmán, *When Animals Dream*, 98.
32 Graeme Shannon et al., "Effects of Social Disruption in Elephants Persist Decades After Culling," *Frontiers in Zoology* 10, no. 62 (2013): 8.
33 Shannon et al., "Effects of Social Disruption in Elephants," 5.
34 Shannon et al., "Effects of Social Disruption in Elephants," 5–6.
35 Shannon et al., "Effects of Social Disruption in Elephants," 4.
36 Shannon et al., "Effects of Social Disruption in Elephants," 6.
37 Shannon et al., "Effects of Social Disruption in Elephants," 5.
38 Ferdowsian et al., "Signs of Mood and Anxiety Disorders in Chimpanzees," e19855, 2.
39 Liana Y. Zanette, Emma C. Hobbs, Lauren E. Witterick, Scott A. MacDougall-Shackleton, and Michael Clinchy, "Predator-Induced Fear Causes PTSD-Like Changes in the Brains and Behaviour of Wild Animals," *Scientific Reports* 9, no. 1 (2019): 6.
40 Zanette et al., "Predator-Induced Fear," 6.
41 Shannon et al., "Effects of Social Disruption in Elephants," 6.
42 Élisabeth Roudinesco, *Freud: In His Time and Ours*, trans. Catherine Porter (Cambridge, MA: Harvard University Press, 2016), 209.
43 Freud, *Beyond the Pleasure Principle*, 24.
44 Bruce Fink, *The Lacanian Subject: Between Language and Jouissance* (Princeton, NJ: Princeton University Press, 1995), 24.
45 Fink, *The Lacanian Subject*, 25.
46 Fink, *The Lacanian Subject*, 24.
47 Jacques-Alain Miller, *Paradigms of Jouissance* (London Society of the New Lacanian School, 2019), 26.
48 Miller, *Paradigms of Jouissance*, 30.
49 Sigmund Freud, *Civilization and Its Discontents*, trans. James Strachey (New York: W. W. Norton & Company, 1961), 164.
50 Freud, *Civilization and Its Discontents*, 165.
51 Lacan, *Écrits*, 393.
52 Freud, *Civilization and Its Discontents*, 165.
53 André Green, *On the Destruction and Death Drives*, trans. Steven Jaron, ed. Howard B. Levine (London: Phoenix Publishing House, 2023), 92.
54 Lacan, *Écrits*, 696.
55 Lacan, *Écrits*, 696.
56 Lacan, *Écrits*, 371.
57 Jacques Lacan, *The Ethics of Psychoanalysis: The Seminar of Jacques Lacan, Book VII*, ed. Jacques-Alain Miller, trans. Dennis Porter (New York: W. W. Norton & Company, 1992), 58.
58 Sigmund Freud, *Introductory Lectures on Psycho-Analysis*, trans. James Strachey (New York: W. W. Norton & Company, 1966), 404.

59 Lacan, *Four Fundamental Concepts*, 184.
60 Jacques Lacan, "Psychanalyse et médecine," in *Lettres de l'école freudienne I* (Paris: École Freudienne de Paris, 1967), 60.
61 T. R. Johnson, *The Other Side of Pedagogy: Lacan's Four Discourses and the Development of the Student Writer* (Albany: State University of New York Press, 2014), 119.
62 Danny DeVito, dir., *Matilda* (Burbank, CA: TriStar Pictures, 1996).
63 Giuseppe Lorini, Donato A. Grasso, and Andrea Loi, "Are Ants Not Only 'Social Insects', but Also 'Nomic Insects'? In Search of Clues of Normativity in the Ant World," *Behaviour* 161, no. 5 (2024): 340.
64 Lorini, Grasso, and Loi, "Are Ants Not Only 'Social Insects'," 340.
65 Daniel C. Marston and Terry L. Maple, *Comparative Psychology for Clinical Psychologists and Therapists* (Jessica Kingsley Publishers, 2016), 183.
66 Alexander J. German, "The Growing Problem of Obesity in Dogs and Cats," *The Journal of Nutrition* 136, no. 7 (2006): 1940.
67 German, "The Growing Problem of Obesity in Dogs and Cats," 1940.
68 Marston and Maple, *Comparative Psychology for Clinical Psychologists and Therapists*, 190.
69 Lacan, *Four Fundamental Concepts*, 115.
70 Charles Darwin, *The Descent of Man, and Selection in Relation to Sex* (London: John Murray, 1871).
71 Marion Petrie, Tim Halliday, and Carolyn Sanders, "Peahens Prefer Peacocks with Elaborate Trains," *Animal Behaviour* 41, no. 2 (1991): 329.
72 Jacques Lacan, *Desire and Its Interpretation: The Seminar of Jacques Lacan, Book VI*, ed. Jacques-Alain Miller, trans. Bruce Fink (Cambridge: Polity Press, 2019), 129.
73 Lacan, *Écrits*, 579.
74 Lacan, *Écrits*, 581.
75 Lacan, *Écrits*, 595.
76 Lacan, *Écrits*, 614.
77 Lacan, *Desire and Its Interpretation*, 214.
78 Walt Whitman, *Leaves of Grass* (Bantam Classics, 2007), 50.
79 Lacan, *Desire and Its Interpretation*, 218.
80 Lacan, *Ethics of Psychoanalysis*, 54.
81 Jacques Lacan, *Transference: The Seminar of Jacques Lacan, Book VIII (1960–1961)*, ed. Jacques-Alain Miller, trans. Bruce Fink (Cambridge: Polity Press, 2015), 211.
82 Lacan, *Transference*, 211.
83 Lacan, *Transference*, 212.
84 Lacan, *Transference*, 212.
85 Lacan, *Transference*, 213.
86 Lacan, *Transference*, 213.
87 C. Lloyd Morgan, *An Introduction to Comparative Psychology* (London: Walter Scott, 1894), 53.

Part 2

Animal Surplus

The Unconscious and Love

Chapter 4

Who Is the Idiot?

Towards an Animal Unconscious

We've discovered, in the foregoing chapters, two stratums of the Other: The symbolic Other (the Other of humanity) and the imaginary Other (the Other of animality). Both these Others adhere to a binding operation in the respective subjects, with the subject adapting themself to the gaze which issues from the 'field of the Other.' However, concluding the analysis here would be premature—it would omit a crucial delineative tenet of the Other, leaving it unanchored from the essential site it issues from. For Lacan, the Other is the place of the unconscious and the Other cannot be fully understood unless it is recognized as such. Lacan famously declares in *Écrits* that "*the unconscious is the Other's discourse*"[1] and locates the Other as the "*unconscious*" site of desire in his formula, "*man's desire is the desire of the Other*."[2] For humans, these declarative formulas have a strict meaning: Human desire is dictated by the Other (the locus of the symbolic where language as a 'site of speech' confronts the subject in their very interiority), and the Other issues from the unconscious, the ineffable strata where its imposition over human desire emanates from.

To provide a straightforward example: Consider the human child's entrance in the symbolic order (gaining access to language via speech). How do their desires come to be? Are we to merely reduce all desire to genetic predisposition or predetermined neurological configurations or instinctive activity? First, for a desire to even be articulated (to participate in a transsubjective communicative gesture), it must be issued through language. The desire must be issued through the Other—refracted by the linguistic universe of signifiers, which is utterly alien and foreign to the child (in the strictly Lacanian lexicon, the *demand* for a *need* is refracted through language in all its non-individuated alterity and the surplus generated is *desire* itself). Lacan writes that "using signifiers transforms the way this need manifests itself . . . what is signified is something beyond raw need and is remodeled through the use of signifiers."[3] Human need, when submitted through the symbolic field, is no longer "raw need," instead "manifesting" as demand which is "fundamentally insoluble."[4] This foreign site—the Other—structures desire through all the unconscious associations related to the signifiers employed in the articulation of demand. Lacan's famous, and to some, enigmatic, aphorism ("man's desire is the desire of the Other") holds a precise meaning in relation to the unconscious, language, and desire: The human subject's desire ("man's desire") is ordered and

DOI: 10.4324/9781003635383-7

unified by the Other of language (ordered by Law), embedded in the unconscious and its censored wishes ("the desire of the Other").

Further, to complicate and inject an additional dimension of everyday reality, take a familial-semantic example—say that a child, a boy, is born into their father's name—they are a junior. Does this act of language, benignly applied to the child and totally in the absence of the child's input or active pre-participation, not function nonetheless to structure their desire? And are these effects of the signifier and the Other—of the name and the language this name is derived from—not maintained in the unconscious and turn out to inform the central meaning of desire? Will the child not either strive to deny or fulfill whatever nominal prophecy comes with this practice of lineage-naming, and will this negation or affirmation not function in relation to a signifier (the name)? Bearing the father's name does construct a pliable linguistic pre-determinism which the child responds to (affirming or negating it are both, of course, responses to something preceding the child-as-agent, namely, the paternal name which preexists the child). The Other—language itself—in its unconscious dimension, determines something essential about the human subject. A symbolic chain—an intersubjective (and intra-subjective) linking of signifiers—governs the subject's desire; for Lacan, humans are "caught up in a symbolic chain" that is "prior to his birth and beyond his death."[5] The signifier's effects, determinative of the subject's 'very being,' are not restricted by the subject and their subjectivity; they only enter a symbolic field that precedes them and exit it—the chain being interminable (as long as subjects exist to prop it up) and the subject being terminable and conspicuously impermanent.

The crucial insight is exactly this: the language which defines the human subject (the totality-lexicon that constitutes a given language as such) is a point of absolute alterity for the subject; yet, in order for the subject to be located and individuated, they must rely on the utter alterity of language to situate their own desire. For the human subject, the Other occupies a paradoxical position of internality and alterity—the Other defines the subject—and the subject may make (literally) nominal contributions to this Other in a marginal, abstract manner (such as creative interventions in language usage), but the Other remains radically distinct from the pre-posited site of the subject's inner-self dominated by consciousness. The Other is both alien and personal—it is the locus of unconscious activity, the foreign place where one feels they *are not*, but paradoxically the site that orients and structures the subject.

While the Other certainly does not operate for animals in the same manner, due to their unavailability to the signifier and human language, it does assist us in delineating a fundamental function of the Other which cannot merely be elided. Crucially, these Lacanian insights remind us that the Other is irreducible to an abstracted structural gaze (as outlined in Chapter 2 on the imaginary) since it must, according to Lacan's very definition of the Other, reside in the unconscious. At this juncture, one can see the impossible bedrock, an unresolved tension, acting as a theoretical surface of inexplicable inscrutability: the possibility of an animal unconscious. We cannot theorize an Other of animality without similarly contending with an unconscious in which the imaginary Other resides. Psychoanalysis is founded on the Freudian 'discovery' of the unconscious, and psychoanalytic insights into animal interiority must contend with the unconscious kernel belying all behavior. However, as we are reminded by the 'authentic' Lacanians, for Lacan, the unconscious is bound up with the symbolic and the function of the signifier; Lacan famously states that "the unconscious is structured like a language," by which he means "the compositional laws of the unconscious, exactly match some of the most fundamental laws of discourse."[6] Bruce Fink explains quite plainly in *The Lacanian Subject* that, according to Lacanian thought, "*the unconscious is* language, meaning that language is that which makes up the unconscious."[7] For Lacan, the signifier is the sole vessel through which the unconscious emerges:

> I am not haphazardly taking the risk of tying [the unconscious] so desperately to the letter, for it is through the mark of arbitrariness characteristic of the letter that the extraordinary contingency of accidents that give the unconscious its true face can be explained.[8]

Emissions of the unconscious—parapraxis, jokes, dreams, typographical errors—can all only be understood as the deployment of unconscious thoughts via the materiality of the signifier and its "arbitrariness." In Lacanian thought, the unconscious can only be conceptualized in terms of language.

Fink illustrates that Lacan also attributes this view to his antecedent Freud, through his notion of the vorstellungsrepräsentanz, translated by Lacan as "representatives of (the) representation."[9] What is repressed are not instincts, drives, or feelings themselves, but rather the *representations* of those impulses—in short, the human unconscious relies on language because the content that is repressed is not actual instincts or drives but language, which is representative of those instincts. Does this psychoanalytic tradition of conceiving of the unconscious in terms of language not mean, as a necessary consequence, the animal has no unconscious? Because the defining demarcation of animality and humanity is access to the symbolic and a 'proper' language-as-language (a language which relies on the signifier) must we not preclude animals from an unconscious? When considering these objections (the exact objections that have led to a unanimous, already-presupposed and unquestionable prejudice against the concept of an animal unconscious), one must recall that the unconscious Lacan is referring to is an unconscious for the human—only for the human is the unconscious 'structured like a language.' This does not automatically grant the animal an unconscious (neither does it preclude them from one)—the unconscious Lacan formulated is merely a strictly human iteration. Lacan is the one, of course, who left available a dimension of the Other for animals, with his insistence that "this is not to say for all that that there is no dimension of the Other with a capital O for the animal."[10]

An animal unconscious does, though, present the theorist with some critical, ostensibly intractable difficulties: The human unconscious—already (wrongly) contested by contemporary positivism—is historically and definitionally disclosed through speech. The unconscious, since the genesis of psychoanalysis with Freud, has been predicated on its emergence through language and, with Lacan's later theoretical intervention, the unconscious is thought to emerge specifically through the signifier's emission via speech and language. In psychoanalytic thought, and specifically Lacanian psychoanalysis, the unconscious can only be known through the signifier's causal 'effects'—the unconscious gains intelligibility through speech.

An animal unconscious presents, then, a dual challenge to the psychoanalytic conception of an unconscious: (1) Animals (those with no access to abstract signifiers as abstract-signifiers—i.e. the animals, besides humans, who only access the sign and whose consciousness is structured by the imaginary register) categorically cannot, according to the conventional psychoanalytic conception of the unconscious as a 'effect' of the signifier, have an unconscious. (2) Despite the—quite compelling and logically coherent—objection that the conventional psychoanalytic rendering of the human unconscious presents, there is a secondary (but much more pragmatic and truly challenging) objection: If there was an animal unconscious, informed, let's say, by the imaginary register, there would be no medium of transmission (as there is for the human unconscious, with the signifier being its medium and grounding—the manner through which the unconscious is transmitted and intelligible; the signifier, of course, not only structures the unconscious but grants it a glimmer of knowability) and due to this mediumlessness, an animal unconscious remains, theoretically and epistemically, ineffable. In short, regardless of the veridicality of an animal unconscious in a phenomenological or theoretical sense, the concept of an unconscious of animality remains replete with lingering epistemic problematics around its knowability—the unconscious *could be* a latent process informing animal behavior and thought, yet its epistemological status, as an overtly and evidentiary *known* phenomenon, is nullified by animals' alienation from the symbolic register. We encounter both an ontological and epistemic problem when theorizing an animal unconscious. Humans would have no access to the dimension of the animal unconscious, like we have to other humans' unconscious processes through the intersubjectively detectable discursive emissions. Dale Jamieson, however, while discussing the apparent inaccessibility of animal thought (consciousness, not unconsciousness), re-formulates the dilemma:

> The problem that we face is not to evade some supposed inconsistency . . . but rather to resolve the unease that arises from the conjunction of our confident commitment to the view that animals think and our apparent ignorance about what it is that they think.[11]

The issue is not that we must gain access to animal conscious thought—let alone an animal unconscious—instead, we must "resolve the unease" that emerges when we realize animals have thought (both conscious and unconscious) *despite* its unavailability to us. I do not proffer in this chapter what is plainly epistemically impossible—perfect knowledge of an animal's thoughts—instead I offer the structure of that thought: not its content transparently-objectively available but its necessary compositional fabric of subjectivity.

The initial objection, on the historical and conceptual propagation of the unconscious as contingent on language-usage (albeit not a frivolous contention), can be cast aside by the following reminder: These conceptions of the unconscious, as stated before, are of the *human unconscious*. When Lacan makes a statement on *the* unconscious, he is merely referring to the only unconscious within the scope of his clinical psychoanalytic experience: the human subject's unconscious. It is certainly true, if one restricts oneself to the human subject, that the unconscious is an effect of the signifier and language, but it is equally true that an animal unconscious—if one accepts it 'ex-ists'—would operate in new, previously unexplored, bounds and could not be apprehended through the prism of language-usage, speech, and the symbolic. An animal unconscious would, instead, reside in the stratum of the scopic-visual field—the imaginary—and adhere to totally distinct regulatory psychic mechanisms tethered to the image, the gaze, and the entire sensory network of the imaginary. In an earlier chapter, we founded animal subjectivity on the bedrock of sensory-image: For animals who participate in the visual field (engaging in the specular function, being subjected to the gaze, or both), this domain structures their experience of the world—and consequently an animal unconscious would be grounded in (or more precisely, formulated according to the principles of) the imaginary register.

At this juncture, establishing that the psychoanalytic view of the unconscious conventionally held (particularly in Lacanian psychoanalysis) would not apply to an animal unconscious (and thus they are not precluded, implicitly, from an unconscious), we encounter the second objection of the utter unknowability—even ineffability—of the animal subject's unconscious. Even if one could, using psychoanalytic theory against itself, isolate an unconscious applicable to (certain) animal subjects, it seems impossible to detect its emergence or even substantiate its existence: How could one ever know that the animal unconscious truly 'exists'?

One should recall, before responding to the previous inquiry, that this same problematic applies to the human unconscious—the human unconscious cannot be identified on an MRI scan; there is no positive, material grounding of the unconscious. One cannot point to a region of the brain and say: *There it is, I see the unconscious!* The unconscious is a psychic mechanism only *knowable via its emergence via effects*. Freud articulates this exact defining principle of the unconscious, writing, "As far as their physical characteristics are concerned [of unconscious processes], they are totally inaccessible to us: no physiological concept or chemical process can give us any notion of their nature."[12] The unconscious is irreducible to physicality (though Freud may have been hoping for an eventual discovery of physical or neuronal correlates). However, we must concede that there is a clinical practice, contingent on discursivity—the symbolic—that prompts and examines unconscious emergences from the analysand, and this is a method certainly without precedent in animality.

While I would not pursue a clinical psychoanalytic practice of animality (for both lack of experiential clinical knowledge and for a certain logical-skepticism of a non-linguistic clinical-psychoanalytic practice involving animals), this does not render the animal unconscious a site of non-existence—rather, it renders it a site of mysteriousness and apparent inexplicability (and this is what the unconscious has always been, whether human or non-human). The animal unconscious is not precluded from existing; it is instead a point that acts as an authentic epistemic limit. A method of detailing its emergence would need to exist, and, as of now, no such methodology is known (and, again, I am not sure if pursuing one, at least in the clinical dimension of psychoanalysis, is a worthy intellectual venture). In his famous essay on subjectivity and the phenomenology of bats, Thomas Nagel writes "to deny the reality or logical significance of what we can never describe or understand is the crudest form of cognitive dissonance."[13] The animal unconscious may never be transparently available to us—but that does not mean that we must "deny" its "reality"; it can remain an epistemic site of inaccessibility (since one is unable to penetrate directly into its contents, non-refracted by theoretical assumptions and biases) *and concurrently* be recognized as *something which exists.*

The preceding discussion should not be conflated with an idiotic affirmation through the negative: It is not that the animal unconscious' current unknowability renders its existence as presumed-to-be true. There are well-founded reasons to ground an animal unconscious—namely the evident procedure of an animal imaginary Other—that do not rely on the unknowability of animals' unconscious. To be more precise—it is the case that the conventional reasons psychoanalysis presents *against* the existence of the animal unconscious are obsolete and non-applicable to animality, but this does not affirm the animal unconscious; instead, it provides an unsettled cleavage, an otherwise concealed theoretical aperture, through which the possibility of an animal unconscious arises.

Others have already gestured towards that cleavage—Nathan Snaza, in his article "Animal Unconscious: Three Questions," interrogates the human monopoly on the unconscious and consequently the denial of an animal unconscious. Relying on Elizabeth Wilson's *Gut Feminism*, which seeks to re-locate the unconscious to not only the mind but also the body—specifically the gut—Snaza argues that

> the concept of the unconscious has to be relocated from just the mind (however widely that has been understood) to reckon with how the body thinks in decentered or distributed ways . . . . If the gut is a seat of the unconscious, then its functioning must be discernable in a wide variety of animal bodies that aren't "human."[14]

When applied to a human, I would be reluctant, if not totally outright reject, the notion of a bodily unconscious—since the unconscious is predicated on the symbolic field rather than corporeality, meaning the human gut may have a physiological effect on subjective-affective mood and even behaviors, but it does not constitute an unconscious as defined by psychoanalytic thought (there is no localizable 'seat' of the human unconscious covertly tucked away in an anatomical location); the body can inform the unconscious, but it is not self-same identical with it—yet, we must consider how a bodily unconscious (or a similar concept) *may* be a legitimate notion for the animal. If the human subject is "decentered," but experiences this fragmentary decenteredness as a unitary wholeness due to the function of the self-reflexive ego, we can proceed with a notion of an animal unconscious that is totally decentered, one that defies the pretentions of human subjectivity.

Derrida, in the critique of Lacan catalogued in the preceding chapter, also supplied a template for conceiving of an animal unconscious. He describes in the same section discussing Lacan:

> We are even less concerned with attributing to what Lacan calls "the animal" what he also calls a "subjectivity" or an "unconscious," which would, for example, allow us to put the animal in an analytical situation (even if such analogous scenarios cannot be completely excluded for certain animals, in certain contexts—and if time permitted we could imagine some hypotheses that would refine that analogy.[15]

What does Derrida mean here by "analogous scenarios"? It is the recognition that an animal unconscious would not be identical to the human unconscious but would instead be predicated on its own structural matrix. Derrida is saying that the "analytical situation" which, to some degree, presumes an unconscious and subjectivity, is not a foreclosed possibility for the animal. Again, Derrida reminds us to leave a conceptual opening for animality. In the preceding chapters, I have sought to develop a theory of animal subjectivity and its relation to Lacan's triadic structure of the symbolic, imaginary, and the Real. In this chapter, I will explore the dimension of the animal subject-beyond-subject—the unconscious and its role in animal interiority—by using the enigmatic apertures provided by theorists such as Lacan and Deleuze. An animal unconscious, like animal subjectivity, can be excavated from Lacan's work through a repudiation of the gesture that collapses humans and animals and an analysis that upholds animal non-negligible specificity. The animal unconscious can only come into frame by de-centering the human unconscious; animal subjectivity must be addressed in its very discordance with human subjectivity.

The Animal Unconscious in the Negative: Repression, Instinct, and the Linguistically-Mediated Drive

The initial partition that putatively precludes animals from an unconscious, aside from the function of language and speech (the domain of the symbolic), is the mechanism of repression. According to Freud, the unconscious forms arising from the repression of material, such as desires or drives, that the conscious cannot contend with—the (temporary) burial of this material to a site inaccessible to consciousness is, definitionally, the unconscious. The unconscious is the graveyard of buried (repressed) material. Lacan, in *Écrits*, explicates the distinctiveness of the Freudian unconscious, illuminating it against the background of other notions, both popular and academic, of the unconscious. He declares that the unconscious is *not* the "the sensory unconscious . . . the automatic consciousness developed by habit . . . the learned and even integrated reserves or memory; the passions in our character which get the better of us; the heredity that is recognized in our natural gifts."[16] The defining characteristic of the unconscious, for the human subject, is the repression of desire due to prohibitions; this is precisely why Lacan declares "the unconscious demonstrates that desire is tied to prohibition."[17] The material of the unconscious is formed by desires that cannot emerge in consciousness because of prohibitions (the symbolic Law) restricting their uninhibited surfacing.

As Juliet Mitchell writes, repression is what grants the Freudian unconscious its conceptually distinctive character—utterly unlike pre-psychoanalytical conceptions that preceded it and those that maintain a cultural presence:

> Until the 1920s the term "unconscious" had been used either loosely, as still it is today in non-psychoanalytic discussions, to describe everything which is not present to consciousness, or more strictly . . . as a mental process, a system in its own right containing all that has been repressed from consciousness . . . within the Freudian unconscious there is a hypothetical area that is always unfathomable and which is produced by what is best known as "primal repression."[18]

Subsequently, that which is repressed later 'tries to push the ideas back into consciousness' by 're-emerging' in a distorted form. Earlier conceptions of the unconscious overlap with the Freudian unconscious insofar as they are referring to material not accessible to consciousness, but in Freudian thought, this is not merely because one fails to apply the spotlight of awareness to the unconscious material—instead, in the Freudian formulation, the unconscious material *cannot* be brought to consciousness (without an intervention through analysis or effort on the part of the subject); the material has a negative gravity in relation to consciousness that expels it, or only releases it in a cryptic, percolative manner, and all this (the productions that the unconscious generates and their opaqueness) is attributable to the mechanism of repression.

To be absolutely emphatic on this point: I am not arguing that animal subjectivity participates in the mechanism of repression and experiences the distortion of unwanted wishes re-emerging at a later time. Nothing in our (limited) understanding of their phenomenology indicates the presence of a censoring force existing in their consciousness. In my conception (which, I believe, aligns with basic Lacanian theory), due to animals lacking a super-ego and the symbolic Law, repression as such cannot occur—it is a foreclosed theoretical possibility. There is no internalized imposition of castration to initiate any repressive activity in consciousness—animals are uncastrated in relation to their desire. On this front, animal consciousness appears more transparent than human consciousness; it seems that there exists no subject-beyond-the-subject and the splitting that Lacan famously assigned to humanity is, in a strict sense, unapplicable to animality. This point should tell us that the animal unconscious, even if only posited in the negative as that-which-it-is-not, is dramatically different from any conception of the human unconscious as postulated by psychoanalysis.

What we are asking when we inquire into the unconscious is effectively this: Which of us (the human and the animals) contain a site of inaccessibility beyond our awareness? *Who does not know—who is the idiot?* Or are we all idiots? The idiot, here defined in the psychoanalytic register as the one who does not know, applies perfectly to the unconscious, that radical site of enigmatic unknowability which leads to an unassailable stupidity in the subject—the site that Lacan defines as "the field of non-knowledge."[19] The unconscious, as the arena of inaccessible self-knowledge that is forever estranged from us, is the ultimate symbol of idiocy. The question, more precisely formulated (since we are already aware that the human is an idiot, insofar as we have an unconscious, rendering our area of consciousness dumbly limited), would actually be: *Is the animal also an idiot? Does the animal share idiot-hood with us?*

It is clear that the animal unconscious cannot be collapsed with the unconscious of humans, but if animals do have something analogous to an unconscious (and the existence of an animal unconscious strikes us as potentially a structural necessity since, otherwise, the imaginary Other would be an unaccountable feature of animal subjectivity without a site of issuance), and a repressive structure does not define the animal unconscious, then how can an animal unconscious be formulated at all? Crucially, Freud in his essay "The Unconscious," indirectly proffers an alternative definition of the unconscious aligning with animal subjectivity:

> The unconscious comprises, on the one hand, acts which are merely latent, temporarily unconscious, but which differ in no other respect from conscious ones and, on the other hand, processes such as repressed ones, which if they were to become conscious would be bound to stand out in the crudest contrast to the rest of the conscious processes.[20]

At play in the definition of the unconscious is both the repressed material, central to psychoanalytic thought, as well as the "latent" unconscious. We have determined that the repressive function is not operative in animality—but the latent unconscious, of that which circulates beneath conscious awareness, remains a viable conceptual schema for apprehending animal interiority (later in this chapter, the "latent" animal unconscious will be carefully demarcated from the instinct-function). Unlike the latent 'temporary' unconscious present in humans, which is unconscious simply because it arises from outside the field of consciousness and the preconscious, we can question whether the latent unconscious of animality "differ in no other respect from" those in consciousness. Is there not a reason certain material, prompting particular behaviors, must remain in the animal unconscious, excluded from a direct confrontation with the realm of consciousness?

A starting, tentative formulation can begin at the notion of splitting—we must begin by situating animality in relation to Lacan's idea of the split subject. Lacan posits the subject is split by the signifier and the field of the Other (which, again, forms the unconscious)—as he explicates in *Écrits*:

> The effect of language is to introduce the cause into the subject. Through this effect, he is not the cause of himself; he bears within himself the worm of the

> cause that splits him. For his cause is the signifier, without which there would be no subject in the real.[21]

The signifier, which is the "effect of language," is the "worm" that "splits" the subject. Lacan confirms this in seminar VII, writing, "It is insofar as the subject is situated and is constituted with relation to the signifier that the break, splitting, or ambivalence is produced in him."[22] What, though, is the subject split between? What are the opposing positions that the subject concurrently occupies? Simply, it is consciousness and the unconscious.

Lacan articulates the relation of this dual split between the conscious and unconscious in the subject—and its relation to language—in his analysis of the subject of the statement and the subject of enunciation. The subject of the statement designates the one who speaks and their speech in its intentionality; it is the conscious deployment of language in its communicative function for a recipient (whether that is another subject in the conventional sense or God—such as the form of a prayer—or even oneself, makes little difference). The subject of enunciation is the betrayal of language, issued through speech, facilitated by the unconscious. The subject of enunciation is the leakage of the unconscious through a communicative act—such as the classic instances of parapraxis or negation or jokes that Freud thoroughly examined in his work. Lacan states that "the presence of the unconscious, being situated in the locus of the Other, can be found in every discourse, in its enunciation."[23] The unconscious is only known through its patterned linguistic emissions—that pattern, or what in Lacan's lexicon is referred to as a structure, *is* the unconscious in humans.

To provide a succinct example of this split in language, consider the polyvalence of a seemingly straightforward statement such as, '*In my dream, I can't recall who I was having intercourse with—but, despite remembering my family being present in the room, it clearly wasn't my mother.*' We detect here a classic case of negation, facilitated by the fundamental split in human subjectivity: That which is asserted as true on the plane of the conscious intentionality of the statement ('it wasn't my mother') is understood to be inverted in the unconscious act of enunciation (*it was my mother*). The function of language, the usage of the Other's alienating alterity to articulate oneself, splits the subject between these two linguistic spheres with their own distinct meaning of speech-acts. One articulates both that which they intend and that which they idiotically do not know that they mean; there is the conscious articulation and the unconscious emission, both using language for their transmission.

Animals are transparently *not* split by the function of the signifier and the symbolic field—it was precisely along these lines that an animal's relation to language was defined as a code or sign rather than a signifier since their communication-acts do not submit to the split between statement and enunciation (and there is no self-referential element of 'speech' to render animals as linguistic subjects). Animals communicate, but they do not use the duplicity of speech. However, despite the Lacanian unconscious—and the split in human subjectivity it engenders—being predicated on language, there is another way to confront this split that may permit room for animality. Bruce Fink explains the Lacanian dichotomy of being and thinking, opposing it to the Cartesian subject:

> The subject, as [Lacan] understands the term, cannot take refuge in an idyllic moment where thought and being coincide but is, rather, forced to choose one or the other. He can 'have' either thought or being, but never at the same time.[24]

Fink describes this as directly antithetical to the Cartesian subject, which consists of a 'one-dimensional self' and an immediate correspondence between thought and being—the Cartesian subject is grounded upon the maxim of 'I think, therefore I am,' while the Lacanian subject is grounded on a more complex formulation of, 'Where I think, I am not.'

Fink tells us that these two disparate conceptions of the subject can be attributed to the Cartesian attachment to the indissoluble ego, "a constructed self taken to be the master of its own thoughts and whose thoughts are believed to correspond to 'external reality.'"[25] Lacan, adhering to the basic Freudian discovery of the psychoanalytic unconscious, instead has his view of subjectivity revolving "around unconscious thought, not the conscious thought studied by Descartes the philosopher."[26] The unconscious is, in human subjectivity, the unaccountable feature that eludes self-reflexive thinking—but it is determinative of being: Where the unconscious is, the subject *is*. Descartes, like all pre-Freudian thinkers, does not consider the being-beyond-thought, which is precisely what Lacan is concerned with and structures his conceptual schema around—for Lacan, being exceeds thought, and when one is thinking, they can be sure that they are not exhausting being. Simply, the Cartesian cogito does not account for the unconscious, the subject-beyond-subject—*the idiot*.

Now, we can sense an opening for an animal unconscious: It is true there is no evidence that animals have the internal material-censoring function of repression, and we have certainly established that animals do not have a direct relation to the signifier and the entire field of the symbolic it constitutes, yet it would appear premature to foreclose the possibility of a split between being and thinking for animality. On what grounds can we definitively assert that animals have no space of interiority that exceeds their thinking? It appears beyond counterintuitive (even unreasonably or fallaciously paradoxical) to posit that thinking and being perfectly coincide across animality. Is the subjective position of animals not ordinarily defined by the proposition that animal being has a non-correspondence to thought—that animals are *not* Cartesian subjects determined by the self-reflexive logic of the cogito? This is precisely what the postulated intellectual hierarchy of beings is predicated on—that humans are rational subjects of the cogito, and animals are irrational subjects devoid of self-reflection.

Presented in a non-hierarchal manner, and inflected by Lacan's insights on subjectivity, we come to a slightly different conclusion than the traditional Cartesian view of animality and humanity: Humans are subjects who *are not where they think* (their unconscious being is exactly where they *cannot* think; humans *are* precisely where conscious thought is *absent*)—yet, of course, this does not posit humans as entirely deficient in thetic self-knowledge: they can think, but the position from which they think (the arena of consciousness) does not exhaust their subjectivity. The animal subject is a subject that can think and, to varying degrees, have self-knowledge (albeit it is non-thetic self-knowledge), but they could not experience the linguistic formulation of *I think therefore I am*. For animals, we can say: *I am, and I think, but I cannot think where I am—I cannot utter 'I am.'* In short, for animals, being overtakes thought—though this is not territory exclusive to the animal (the exact same could be said about humans and their relation to unconscious emissions).

We can unequivocally say—while risking no real substantive contestation from any side of the 'animal question'—that animals have a 'being' inaccessible to 'thought' (animal thought does not reflexively pervade their being, meaning, in the simplest terms, that their actions do not always pass through the screen of thought—animal action and behavior is oftentimes devoid of thought as self-awareness, as is human action and behavior), especially since this is the traditional defining demarcation between humanity and animality. But, while we conceive of this being as embedded in non-thought, which is ratified by psychoanalysis as 'the unconscious' in a human, can we say the same about an animal? There is surely a split in the animal-subject between thought and being—but is the being that defines animal subjectivity, as occupying the arena of non-thought, not merely the subjective space of instincts as opposed to a proper unconscious? Ordinarily, this is precisely what animal being is said to be composed of—the thoughtless space of instinctive sub-subjectivity.

Lacan follows this logic of animal unconscious and animal instinct (founded on the field of the symbolic and the "effect of enunciation" of signifiers), stating:

> [O]ne can illustrate the effect of enunciation by asking a student if he can imagine the unconscious existing in animals, unless they have some degree of language—human language. If he indeed agrees that this is the condition that would allow him to at least consider the possibility, you have verified that he distinguishes between "unconscious" and "instinct."[27]

Here, Lacan clearly attributes the space that occupies the "unconscious" in humans to "instinct" in animals. This demarcation is due, again, to the capacity of "human language" (the symbolic). Yet, one should interrogate Lacan's claim here: What does he mean by "instinct," and why, unlike the human, who has an unconscious (alongside instinct), does instinct entirely exhaust animal being and leave no remainder for an unconscious to occupy? From this point, rather than pursuing strict fidelity to Lacan's conception of animal interiority, we must explore the limits of his articulation of animal subjectivity, to re-orient it or re-contextualize it—if we must, we will conceptually and epistemically stretch Lacanian thought to meet new coordinates beyond his focus on human psychoanalysis to develop true zoological psychoanalysis.

What does Lacan mean by instinct—and how are instincts distinguishable from his conception of the drive? Lacan writes explicitly that, "[t]he drive, as it is constructed by Freud on the basis of the experience of the unconscious, prohibits psychologizing thought from resorting to 'instinct.'"[28] Elsewhere, in Seminar XI, he asserts the same principal distinction: "trieb [drive] and instinct have nothing in common . . . . Trieb gives you a kick in the arse, my friends—quite different from so-called *instinct.*"[29] Although humans have both instincts and drives, for Lacan, animals only have instincts and no drives—as we saw, he even relies on the concept of instincts to deny that an animal unconscious exists. Lacan's provides a relatively simple explication of instincts and drives for the human in *The Ethics of Psychoanalysis*: "the instinct is the effect of the mark of the signifier on need, their transformation as an effect of the signifier into something fragmented and panic-stricken that we call the drive."[30] Here, Lacan immediately identifies instinct and drive in a triangulation with the signifier's "effect": the instinct is caused by "need" (an instinct is activated by the gravity of a being's bio-needs); however, for humans, the instinct is filtered through the function of the signifier, thereby generating a new response devoid of need—and this is the function of the drive and its site of emergence. To a scrupulous reader of Freud, something is surely conspicuously at odds between the Freudian and Lacanian account of instincts and drives: Freud employs, in the English translation, the term "instinct" for precisely what we are calling "drive" (for instance the death drive)—an impulse beyond need. Lacan clarifies that, in the original German texts, two terms are used: *trieb* (drive) and *instinkt* (instinct), which are, upon translation by James Strachey (who translated Freud's work into English), united into one word that conflates the meaning of both terms—the word in English being 'instinct.'

Again, like the function of desire in humans, the formal equation of drive can be understood according to the subtraction of need following instinct's submission to the signifier (*desire* is a *demand* issued through the *signifier* subtracted by *need*; *drive* is *instinct* issued through the *signifier* subtracted by *need*)—drives, then, are unconscious in origin; they are dispatched from the Other and definitionally exceed any bio-need of the subject. Lacan makes this distinction evident:

> I've no objection to the definition of what may be called instinct, nor even to the customary use of the word, as for example calling the needs that living beings have to feed themselves instincts. But the oral drive is something else.[31]

An instinct is bound by the pleasure principle and bio-need—Judith Roof defines instincts as "an impetus not instigated by an outside stimulus but coming from something already inherent to the body of the organism."[32] Instinct is the biologically auto-mandated gravity that brings one to their mother's nipple to satiate hunger; drive, though it has an originary proximity to needs and instincts, becomes unbound to need and the pleasure principle (causing it to frequently fall into painful beyond-satisfaction jouissance)—the drives propel the human subject to continue sucking when there is no longer a nipple present and despite there being no need that is addressed by the act (like the oral fixation of thumb-sucking—severed from the instinct to satiate hunger by reliance on the nipple, displaced, through drive, onto a new object). As is evident, this sucking no longer serves a function toward satiating a bio-need: It offers something (as the object of the drive) that the subject returns to again and again, with the subject reaching for its Real jouissance.

Undoubtedly, animals are guided by instincts: The instincts orient an animal's subjectivity around needs (sustenance, reproduction, safety)—and there is nothing in the behavior of animals that indicates the presence of a human-like, linguistically-structured drive. Lacan does not, however, condemn animality to absolute fidelity to instinctual activity—he actually relies on animals as an example of how the imaginary field transcends instinct: "Images as such have a captivating character beyond their corresponding instinctual mechanisms, as is shown in both sexual and combative animal display."[33] The structural vortex of animal subjectivity, meaning the imaginary register—contingent on the image-of-another—is not bound to instinct; there is an instinct exceeding pure instinct, namely through "display." As we saw with the peacock's *display*, the animal-image (and the image animals have of another) are not bound to instinct—the image produced (the colorful display) has no direct relation to bio-need, though it may, in the end, serve a reproductive function.

Even if Lacan is clear that animals—and the imaginary field—are not limited to instinctual activity, we must qualify the concept of instinct: Instinct does not necessarily mean animals are mechanistic. In some animals, such as insects, this may be the case, but in others, particularly social mammals, the thrust of instinct and its structuring procedure cannot be limited to a pure machine-like input-output. Paul Katsafanas writes that instinct is totally distinct from a mechanistic subject devoid of choice and authentic subjectivity:

> I think we can see well enough why mechanistic explanations of instinct seem problematic: it's hard to envision what the mechanistic processes driving complex, temporally extended, goal directed courses of activity would be. It's also easy to see why instinctive activities can't be treated as fully conscious activities: while we might say that these actions involve awareness of certain proximate goals, the organism has no awareness of the distal goal that is served by these proximate ones. The wasp may know that it is collecting grubs and so on; but it cannot know that it is storing these grubs near its eggs so that the larvae that it will never see will have a nourishing meal. Moreover, the entire stretch of activity is unlearned, yet performed perfectly the first time it is done. Conscious direction can't be required here.[34]

Instincts are neither "mechanistic" nor "conscious" in animality—the goals they are directed towards exceed this view. However, despite the fact that instincts are more complicated than they initially appear, instinctual activity cannot be said to be unconscious in a psychoanalytic sense. This is where we must appeal to drives. Drive as linguistically-mediated is certainly outside the bounds of animality—but we should ask ourselves at this juncture: Are all of animals' behaviors oriented perfectly towards pure bio-need? Are there no superfluous behavioral directions—meaning those that exceed, or even explicitly undermine, *need*—that what we would refer to as the animal 'instinct' pulls them?

On this point, there is an aperture, a conceptual cleavage for an animal drive: Animal behavior, which is normally theoretically reduced to instinct, is empirically not delimited by *need* (the many examples of animal jouissance enumerated in the preceding chapter exhibit exactly this). On this front, there are two, somewhat mutually exclusive, approaches to pursue the question of animal instincts and their relation to need and drive: One could reasonably object that all animal behavior not directed towards a need is an evolutionary misfire—that it ultimately *is* oriented towards need but that the orientation has, for some unknown and potentially undiscoverable reason, been diverted from need's path, either through a biological mis-configuration or some other undiscovered means. Take the example, derived from Chapter 2 on the imaginary, of imperfect mimicry in animals: Imperfect mimicry—a misconfiguration between the putatively advantageous mimetic behavior, development, or evolutionarily formed attribute of an animal and the object being mimicked (such as a smaller animal mimetically issuing the sound of a larger animal to feign a predatorial status—but there being a sonic severance between the sound issued and the authentic predatorial sound) leading to an evolutionary disadvantage or net neutral advantage—does not necessarily indicate that mimicry's function is aimed at something other than need.

In short, what appears to be animal drive, oriented towards some non-need, is actually (according to the 'misfire' interpretation) a distorted instinct—an instinct whose end remains need even if its execution does not ultimately bring a given animal into closer proximity with that end. It seems reasonable to ascertain that many features of animality which serve non-need could be understood as mis-tincts (improperly aligned or executed instincts). However, we should not automatically grant this view of drives as pure mis-tincts: Could the same reductive evolutionary perspective not also be applied to human drives—where all drives become circumstantially deformed instincts? Consider, again, the example of the oral fixation that finds the object of the thumb. Can the displaced fixation on the thumb not be considered an 'evolutionary misfire' which misses its proper object, instead landing on an object that serves no purpose in terms of survival or bio-need? This interpretation, if taken seriously, could attempt to explain all drives as improperly executed instincts—but psychoanalytic practice tells us that the drive is not a misapplied instinct; it is, instead, a behavior that diverts from need, acting as a surplus need, generating a domain separate from that of instinct.

Another explanation for the apparent severance-divorce between need and behavior in animality could be the existence of a proper, non-linguistically mediated drive in animality: an authentic drive towards an aim which exceeds (or even directly undermines) bio-need. Where do we see this most clearly with the animal if not the death drive? Freud, in his seminal essay "Beyond the Pleasure Principle," identifies the contesting force against self-preservation in animality: a movement towards distinctly ill-adaptive repetition and regression—even going so far as to detect this impulse in all organisms: "*It seems, then, that an instinct is an urge inherent in organic life to restore an earlier state of things.*"[35] Later, he calls this restorative regression to an earlier state the "first instinct" for the primordial life-form—meaning that upon the emergence of life itself, in whatever form that may have been, there was "the instinct to return to the inanimate state"[36]—he even explicitly states that "*the aim of all life is death.*"[37] Further, he acknowledges the conceptual discontinuity that the "death drive" presents to the theory of instincts: The instincts, as we've seen, are conceived as "impelling towards change and development, whereas we are now asked to recognize in them, the precise contrary—an expression of the *conservative* nature of living substance."[38] Freud then provides apt examples from animality, precisely to show that the drive he is describing is not limited to humans and has Darwinian continuity to other non-human species; Freud seeks to show that the drive regressively impelling one towards non-being is embedded in any life-form and accordingly does not somehow appear spontaneously as an aberrative rupture in the human species. The drive causes repetitive behavior in animality, with Freud providing examples from fish and birds:

> When certain fish undertake arduous journeys at spawning-time, in order to deposit the spawn in certain definite waters far removed from their usual habitats, according to the interpretation of many biologists they are only seeking the earlier homes of their kind, which in course of time they have exchanged for others. The same is said to be true of the migratory flights of birds of passage . . . in the phenomena of heredity and in the facts of embryology we have the most imposing proofs of the organic compulsion to repetition.[39]

Freud detects in the "organic compulsion to repetition" the ratification for his notion of the drive-beyond-instinct: The fact that animal behavior, that we would otherwise designate as 'instinctual,' sought to restore an earlier stage with no import regarding survival (possibly even accentuating the likelihood of survival due to the energy expended in the "compulsion to repetition") means that there are two classes of compulsory behavior in animals; animals have both drive and instinct.

In Judith Roof's article on Freud's use of microscopic Protista (which are, oftentimes, uni-cellular), she explains that he relied on these 'simpler' and earlier forms of life to demonstrate that the antagonism between instinct and drive is always present—from the putatively 'lowest' to the 'highest' beings. Roof explains that Freud "regards" the splitting of germ-cells "as the primal moment of reproduction and the sexual instinct."[40] This interpretation was reasonable to Freud because, similar to how sexual reproduction seeks to 'preserve' the animal who engages in it (through the transmission of one's DNA over generations), germ-cells splitting also "exist to preserve the germ-cell."[41] Roof also exhibits how Freud not only attributed instincts to uni-cellular organisms but also (death) drives: Freud detects "a death instinct in the single celled organism's primal living matter."[42] Because the single celled organism eventually capitulates to senescence, there is a 'natural' drive back towards the inorganic state of non-life from the very start of animated life. Freud here takes his claim that "aim of all life is death" to its absolute conclusion—applying it to even the unicellular organism. This is essential to understanding Freudian instinct and drive because since

> [t]he unicellular character of the protista example suggests that the forces that govern their behavior must be intrinsic to cell matter itself, and if intrinsic to the cell, which comprises life, then it is intrinsic to all life as well.[43]

Roof articulates her reservations about the veracity of Freud's claims, writing that "single celled organisms" are "flexible enough"[44] to lead to his desired theory of a contesting life-instinct and death-drive—insinuating that Freud was willing to use protista as an example despite the biological truth-value of the assertions. The point here, though, is not (only) the biological evidence underpinning Freud's claim, but rather that animality—even in its simplest cellular form—is implicit in Freud's conception of instincts and drives.

André Green, relying on work by the biologist Jean Claude Ameisen, does argue explicitly that there is scientific veridicality of the death drive in the functioning of the cell:

> One after another, the division which engenders the multitude [of cells], the differentiation whence is born diversity and migration (the movement of cells throughout the body), punctuates each stage. In parallel are produced 'natural' disappearances, a disconcerting discovery having to do with a mysterious cause. What's the purpose of these deaths? Here's the answer: "The deconstruction of the body, as it builds itself, is one of the essential components of the development of complexity" (Ameisen, 1999, p. 30).[45]

At a cellular level, destruction (death) is the result of "complexity"—and one could detect here the basic insight of entropy: the implacable deterioration over time of material and energy. Attributing this to entropy—the process of death itself—would be false. Ameisen is not merely asserting cells deteriorate over time; the true kernel is that the cells die due to "self-destruction," which Ameisen unflinchingly refers to as "cell-suicide."[46] As Green writes, "cell death was programmed"[47]—within the cell, with its supposedly singular focus on propagation and self-preservation, there is an embedded prearrangement for self-death. Green relies on cell-suicide to prop up the death drive against the background of scientism, which has long insisted on the 'impossibility' of the death drive. The cell's nature informs us of a drive-toward-death on the cellular level.

At this juncture, a reader can likely preemptively anticipate my explanation for the gap between Lacan's definition of drive as linguistically-mediated and Freud's (and others') examples of a drive in animality (even at the level of uni-cellularity) that is detached from language: Lacan's delineation of drive is intended to exclusively illuminate the procedure of the human drive. Lacan was, of course, a psychoanalytic clinician (and occupied a status as a prominent teacher of other clinicians and theorists during his seminars), and his goal was the illumination of *human* psychic processes. While Lacan's intervention was crucial in describing the severance between instinct and drive, bio-need, and compulsion-beyond-need, he did inadvertently elide the place of drive in animality—instead relying on the classic distinction between language and languagelessness—human and animal—to define the operations of drive and need. The next step, then, in approaching the contours of an animal unconscious is a proper disquisition on animal drives that does not efface previous psychoanalytic discussions but instead acts as a functional theoretical extension. Lacan and Freud are not incorrect on the drive and instinct—they are only guilty of not taking the concepts far enough beyond the human.

The Idiot and the Other: Animal Death Drive, PredaOther, and Dreams

Animal drives can be understood from multiple vantages, but the death drive, as the destructive compulsion to repeat—the striving towards the inanimate—offers the most explicit opposing pole to need, instinct, and its structural grounding, the pleasure principle. In Freud's words, the death drive could be defined as the "circuitous paths to death" that "present us to-day with the picture of the phenomena of life."[48] To make sense of the "phenomena of life," with all its attendant multidirectionalities (appearing nonsensical, on the surface, in evolutionary terms), can only be understood through appeal to a death drive. The death drive is, of course, countered by the drive towards self-preservation that need, and sexual activity, presents—which, in conjunction with the death drive, provide a "picture" of the operation of life. We detect the death drive present in all self-destructive symptoms clinically plaguing humans and even the pull, in a certain subset of humanity, towards melancholic suicidality (if the melancholic-suicidal subset can even be coherently demarcated from the whole of humanity—it remains to be seen if humanity as a totality does not sense, either dully or powerfully, this pull-towards-death. Does the death drive not implicitly pervade all human behavior?). Can there truly be a similar argument for animality? Can animality be said to have a 'death drive,' or are the behaviors which seem to mirror the death drive only aberrative regressions? Does a true death drive—like we detect in humanity—not necessitate a higher order of consciousness? Again, to refer to the Lacanian split: The death drive relies not on higher order consciousness, but rather idiocy, meaning, in a psychoanalytic account, not a lack of intelligence, but the presence of an inaccessible region of subjectivity in an a-spatial sense—an unconscious—which leads to a directionality that defies the need-fulfilling instinct. Since, as André Green writes, "The death drive, after all is said and done, is suicidal,"[49] we must begin explicating the death drive by first exploring suicidality in animals.

In an article titled "The Suicidal Animal," Edmund Ramsden and Duncan Wilson offers a careful historical reading of scholarship on animal suicidality, enumerating the vacillating intellectual and cultural discourse on the subject. Ramsden demonstrates that, in the 1800s, animal suicide is postulated as a "largely rational act,"[50] ratifying Darwin's claims on a continuity between animality and humanity, and he finds that human-animal continuity was rhetorically employed by early associations for animal welfare. This view was corroborated by anecdotal instances of animal deaths and informed, partially, by romantic notions of animal suicide as a corollary of human courage and individuality. Lord Byron's scorpion from his poem *The Giaour* is, as Ramsden and Wilson explains, exemplary of the rationality presupposed in animal suicide as well as the assertion's reliance on anecdotal information: In the poem, itself a retelling of earlier folklore, the scorpion chooses to "cure all pain" (via 'suicide'—i.e. stinging their own bodies) when they are "girt by fire."[51] Later, in the "scientific" age of animal experiments, the scorpion suicide is re-capitulated as "self-destruction";[52] Conway Lloyd Morgan, after conducting experiments with scorpions, subjecting them to unbearable conditions that induce the self-stinging behavior, concluded that the self-sting was not "a conscious act of suicide" and should be interpreted plainly as an auto-reflexive behavioral response. (Morgan's interpretation adheres, of course, to his famous canon that sanctions a lower-order reading of animal consciousness and behavior.)

Subsequently, ethologists and animal psychologists in the 20th century conducted empirical animal experiments and centered their understanding of animal self-destruction around the concept of "stress": "emotions of rage and fear, necessary for 'fight or flight', could, if severe, have destructive effects on the nervous system."[53] These responses were all engendered by instances of extreme stress. Here, we detect a classification applicable to both humans and animals: the self-destructive response provoked by immense, utterly unbearable stress. However, this is surely distinct from suicidality as a 'conscious' intentional act—apprehension of finitude and mortality must, we are told, accompany authentic 'human' suicidality. Ramsden and Wilson cite a psychiatrist named Ivor Jones who disclaims the legitimacy of suicide as an exclusively human act:

> [D]epression in most suicides probably impairs the capacity for rational thought while at the same time inducing suicide impulses. We suggest that suicide may be a uniquely human attribute only because our definition of it makes it so; in other words, if suicide were to be defined as a destructive act inflicted on the self leading to death, then animal analogies do exist.[54]

In short, suicide (defined as an act which requires conscious intentionality) is only conceived in this manner to delineate human suicide as such, to the exclusion of any non-human self-caused death. Suicide is another addition to the litany of attributes deployed to define the tenuous fabric of humanity's self-aware consciousness against a backdrop of its absence in the animate and inanimate beyond us. Despite Jones' intervention, claiming the definition of suicidality is determined by human acts of purposive self-destruction, it still remains true that animals do not engage in the same acts of self-annihilation that humans do. It is telling, though, to dispatch scenarios from the liminal margins of humanness: If a child, with no apprehension of their impermanent finitude and the precariousness of life, kills themselves during an emotional fit, does this not constitute a suicide due to the child's non-apprehension of the truly irrevocable 'consequence' of their actions? What if a fully adult human is subjected to unbearable torture and reflexively kills themselves, is the true causality not aversion of pain, overtly analogous to the scorpion's self-sting, rather than a self-aware intentionality to detach oneself from the finitude of life? Further, can we not recognize here a metaphor for depression: Does one not kill themselves when they are depressed as a way of eluding unbearable pain? Is it the case that the depressed person does not want to live, or rather, that they have a biological duty, at any cost, to avoid the extreme pain of depression? This cannot be said to serve the instinct for the perpetuation of life, and while it would certainly be said to issue from the death drive, it is also not a clear instance of suicidal intentionality. Does the depressive in psychic-melancholic pain, who kills themselves, *not* commit suicide?

Whether or not a self-induced animal death can be designated as suicide, it is the death of oneself (or even harm-towards-death) caused by oneself (self-annihilation) which situates animals in the death drive. The death drive is not necessarily bound to intentional suicide. Ramsden and Wilson reference the psychoanalyst Karl A. Menninger's book *Man Against Himself*, which delineates the death drive as an "innate, unconscious and destructive drive" which is "common to all and, when aggressive and destructive impulses found no outlet, it underlay a variety of self-destructive behaviors."[55] The death drive is "a more general self-destructive impulse" including a range of behaviors such as "self-starvation, dehydration and the refusal of medical treatment (organic), accidents, dangerous sports and smoking (chronic suicide), and self-mutilation (partial and focal suicide)."[56] While Menninger is not referring to animals or propagating a theory of the death drive in animality, the pertinence to animal behavior is quite transparent: The death drive is not isolated to suicidality—it encompasses the entire broad range of self-destructive behaviors, and animals undoubtedly participate in some of these behaviors. Did we not, in the preceding chapter on animal jouissance, demarcate an animal drive to self-effacement via an enjoyment-beyond-pleasure? When the animal eats-towards-death, are they not eliding the instinct to preserve life towards some other end—emanating from another drive?

Additionally, the death drive accounts for animal anorexia: It is an ethological fact that there are animals who experience a destructive lack-of-hunger. As researcher Jeong Won Jahng demonstrates in a 2010 study on rat maternal separation and eating disorders, rats who are deprived of their mother for sustained periods, during crucial infant developmental stages, experience anhedonia—the reduction in pleasure or enjoyment. This leads to "reduced intake of palatable food during adolescent period . . . in accordance with previous report showing decreased consumption of palatable food in an animal model of depression."[57] To proffer a summation in terms of clinical eating disorders: the fact of being "removed from their dam and home cage"[58]—meaning, crucially, they were separated from their mothers—led to temporary depressive symptoms such as anorexia (though these symptoms seemed to be offset over time, normally leading to a comparable body weight to the rats who were not subjected to maternal separation). We should detect, in this fact of fleeting adolescent animal anorexia (caused not by physical injury, but instead by depression—a subjective, experiential condition), an instance of the death drive merely refracted through a new route: The same drive that propels eating-towards-death accounts for diminution-of-pleasure (anhedonia) and refusal-of-eating (anorexia). One must recognize the utter radicality of this—if animals are thought of as instinctual machines whose existence functions solely towards self-presentation, particularly on the level of a rat, then the fact of an animal experiencing anhedonia (an utterly anti-instinctual operation), informs us of an underlying drive; in animals, there is a tentacular drive towards death, circulating through the animal and escaping through disparate means.

Self-destruction, of course, is not limited to jouissance—jouissance is not a precondition for causing one's own death: the death drive unconsciously meanders through numerous behavioral passages, erupting in lethal and non-lethal effusions. These ruptures, all directing the animal subject against the otherwise life-sustaining gravity of self-preservation, and the underlying formation governing their reversed, anti-life directionality, are indicative of a source beyond manifest consciousness—a structure latently functioning below the immediate surface, namely an animal unconscious.

If instincts anchor animal behavior in self-preservation and life itself, then the death drive inverts the anchor of life, instead grounding animal behavior in the inexorable pull towards the original 'inanimate state' that Freud claims all life is indirectly oriented towards. However, a behavior is strictly defined as instinctual only if it bypasses cognition: An instinct is opposed to reflective action in humans by its non-submission to thetic-reflective cognition. Why, then, are instincts not designated as unconscious in animality? Why does the death drive act as an entry-point to the animal unconscious when the instinct, much more apparently accessible and on the behavioral surface, remains relegated to consciousness in animality? These issues are compounded by the fact that, in humans, instincts unequivocally are constitutive (at least partially) of the unconscious: instincts (or to be precise, their representation captured by signifiers) are repressed and contribute to the unconscious's structural constitution. Conversely, in animality, there is no representational construction of the instinct, only its phenomenological gravity.

The classic Freudian Oedipus complex demonstrates the place of instinct in unconscious formation: there is an early sexual instinct directed at a parent-object that is subsequently repressed, resulting, later in life, in the well-known inadvertent and cryptic emissions undermining the conscious intentionality of the subject—the displacement of parent and spouse in speech or the revealing joke eluding the limited grasp of consciousness. Without addressing the limits of the Oedipus complex as a psychoanalytic theory, we can ascertain the fundamental insight: Human instinct (particularly the sexual instinct) is behavior liable to inform the unconscious—for animals, this is not the case. If an animal unconscious can be asserted to exist, it cannot be founded on the basis of instinct due to the absence of repression in animality—human repression is what converts the economic life-libido of instincts into material for the unconscious. Conversely, the death drive must, definitionally, elude consciousness: The Death drive, as the utter polarity of life's putative end (from a biological perspective), which is the perpetuation of life both individually and reproductively, operates covertly beneath conscious awareness, emerging in the disparate unconscious emissions which Menninger (following Freud) enumerated.

Consider the symptoms delineated in the preceding chapter on deadly jouissance—such as the jouissance of obesity which domesticated animals exhibit—is this not the perfect instantiation of the death drives and its underlying thrust to return to an inanimate state? Or even Lord Byron's 'suicidal' scorpion—which subsequently becomes a proper object of science and is determined to commit the self-terminating act ascribed by folk tales—if the animal subject is oriented solely towards the activating pull of life, then how would the scorpion's self-caused death be a rational possibility? We see, in both these instances, emblematic examples indicative of an anti-life drive—a death drive. Yes, instinct may be the prevailing force in the subjective economy of an animal, but the death drive is a subversive force also present in the wide-ranging self-destructive symptoms.

The singular exception to this would appear to be humanity and the possibility of our purposive orientation towards death in full knowledge of our finitude—suicide brings the death drive into consciousness; suicidality is the subject consciously contending with the death drive in its absolute anti-life radicality. As established, animals do not contend with authentic suicidality—or, at least, they are not equipped with suicidality defined as conscious intentionality of one's own death with a corresponding knowledge of the horizon that death represents to life. Instinct, then, represents the consciousness of animality (due to the lack of a repressive, censoring operation in animal subjectivity) and the (death) drive represents the animal's undetected unconscious. If animals are agents of life—having subjectivity and making choices—they are surely thinking-towards-life, and the non-thought (the unthinkable) is the unconscious orientation towards-death.

Consider, yet again, the theory of Roger Caillois on mimicry: Mimicry is, to him, "depersonalization by assimilation to space."[59] It is a drive towards in-distinction—towards the loss of a subjective entity in their environment. Embedded in Caillois' theory of mimicry is not only the death drive—since the animal seeks to dissolve the bounds constitutive of themself, but also an Other in its two animal variants: The Other and the predaOther. As Lacan demonstrated, the Other is a factor whenever mimicry is enacted in the absence of a predator. Without the presence of an individuated other, such as a predator, who is the mimetic activity *for*? This must be an Other that exceeds all instantiations of (little 'o') others; there must be a predaOther where the gaze issues from beyond all predators. Where does this Other issue from if not the unconscious? They cannot be said to issue outside the animal subject—the predaOther should not be conflated with an-other who is a predator, since the Other is never limited to an (individuated) other (an-other can only be representative of the Other, such as the mOther). The gaze of the Other issues from a site within the subject that is alien to them—the animal subject's Other is not an imaginary accessible place of subjectivity; it is an inaccessible, endogenous space beyond thought that nonetheless informs their behaviors. The Other is the subject-within-the-subject that posits itself from without. A gaze issued from the Other appears under the guise of exogeneity despite its complete internality—like the growl that is posited as outside oneself yet actually issues from one's own stomach. This means the animal unconscious is not exhausted by the death drive. For instance, the predaOther is not related to the death drive: It is squarely consonant with adaptive instinctual behavior to preserve life. Instinct has split itself within the animal subject—into a drive that exceeds bio-need (such as the mimetic response to the predaOther) and a drive that subverts it (such as the explicit symptoms of the death drive). Here we have arrived at the necessary dimension in order for activity to be designated as unconscious in animality—it must emanate from *within* yet posit its activity *exogenously* (since it issues from the Other).

The fact of animal dreams acts as additional evidence to the presence of an animal unconscious. Freud famously discussed the dreams of animality, writing:

> What animals dream of I do not know. A proverb for which I am indebted to one of my pupils professes to tell us, for it asks the question: 'What does the goose dream of?' and answers: 'Of Maize.' The whole theory that the dream is the fulfilment of a wish is contained in these two sentences.[60]

While the animal dream is potentially 'simpler,' it cannot be said to be an effect of thinking—consciousness—even the animal dream is an unconscious effect. Since it is defined by the cessation of conscious activity, the dream can certainly not be considered conscious activity. The animal dream-wish, like the human-dream wish, is an unconscious wish: A goose's wish for maize issues from the unconscious, though (we can guess) in a far less distorted way than the human's ambivalent wish for their loved one's death.

In his book *When Animals Dream*, David M. Peña-Guzman appeals to research that proves "[w]ith a few possible exceptions, all mammals dream . . . . If we look at electrophysiological data, it is likely that birds and fish also dream."[61] Guzman provides countless examples—from birds (zebra finches) whose neural activity while sleeping "was an exact structural replica" of their "singing while awake"[62] to the "hippocampal activity"[63] of rats which demonstrated that they continued to run a track they had started when awake—and thoroughly establishes (despite the insistence, on the part of many scientists to refer to these dreams as visual-spatial 'replays,' preferring to somehow abstract them of any phenomenological experience) that this activity is clearly embodied mental phenomena experienced while the animal is asleep (which is, definitionally, a dream). He later uses the dream life of animals to establish their subjectivity: "any creature who dreams is necessarily subjectively conscious and therefore has a feeling of subjective presence as well as a sense of bodily self-awareness."[64] While I agree that the dream establishes an animal subjectivity, I do not think that the dream can be classified as an activity of the merely conscious subject: *Yes, the dream may be indicative of animal subjectivity, but that does not mean it issues from consciousness*. The nightmare—where the subject undergoes some form of fear-inducing experience—is indicative of the dream-experience as unconscious activity. To return to the example referenced in Chapter 3, Peña-Guzman describes the nightmares of rats who had been tortured by researchers during the day using electrical shocks, writing: "the rats were experiencing nightmares triggered by traumatic memories . . . they would retrieve memories of their not-so-distant past and re-live them in the form of a dream."[65]

Unlike the simple wish-fulfillment of a dream, which seems to correspond to conscious activity, the nightmare introduces new complications. Namely, from what site must these nightmares erupt? Can they simply be said to be the subject 'consciously' reflecting on trauma while asleep? Why would the animal replay their own torture? We must think of this as an imposition from the *without-within*—the animal unconscious. The nightmares are not *actually* imposed exogenously, but they may feel that way to the rat since they issue from a zone of consciousness inaccessible to them. Lacan's refers to nightmares as instances of the "Other's jouissance," writing: "the nightmare's anxiety is felt, properly speaking as that of the Other's jouissance."[66] Yet again, by reflecting on modern animal research and Lacan's statements, we must situate animals in relation to the Other. The nightmare feels as if it is inflicted exogenously—as if it derives from a source outside the subject who rejoices in the pain, when in fact, of course, it is a subjective production from the subject-within-the-subject, the Other. The psychic pain that the rat feels at replaying their torture is experienced as an-other's jouissance—when it is really their own jouissance (via the Other) at approaching the Real beyond pleasure. Again, we catch a glimpse here of a death drive operating beyond the pleasure principle within animality. If animals experience nightmares, then there must be a zone of the Other at play.

What of the Freudian second topology (the so-called 'structural model' consisting of the superego, ego, and the id)? Could we not attribute the jouissance of animality, the death drive, animal nightmares, and the predOther to a frenzied, un-directed id rather than an animal unconscious? It is precisely the dimension of the Other which precludes this interpretation. The id presents itself as an intrinsic impulse (the instincts and id are, of course, closely related if not synonymous), but the unconscious arises from the Other, which feels as if *it were not one's self*. This is the crucial distinction: Yes, the id may be destructive in its 'primitive' deployment of libido, and animal activity may certainly be partly directed by the id, but the id is, definitionally, guided by instincts—there is no Other at play in the id, only the self (instinctual behavior issues from the self—however limited the corresponding sense of self may be, whether reflective or immanent—not the Other). It is not posited, in its phenomenology, as exogenous but rather totally endogenous. Further, while the id may be destructive, it is normally destructive towards others for the self; destruction is activated in the name of self-preservation and pleasure, and self-destruction (when issued from the id) only comes from the consequences of this behavior. The id, understood as such, is partially incommensurate with the function of the death drive for the animal.

While we find—through animal nightmares, mimicry, obesity, and anorexia—an undercurrent of the death drive structuring their subjectivity, issuing from an unconscious that animals tacitly experience, this does not open up the unconscious as an utterly capacious notion to be applied beyond the domain of the living-sentient. A psychoanalytic articulation of an animal unconscious necessitates contending with other non-human entities—if the partition which previously divided animals and humans, historically precluding animals from being conferred a status as psychoanalytic subjects, has been exposed as unfounded, then other forms of 'intelligence' are also legitimately eligible for reappraisal under these same conditions, namely artificial intelligence. If animals, who do not speak (in terms of deploying the signifier—they do, of course, have other communicative transmissions), have an unconscious, then what of AI and its putative intelligence and use of language? Does AI itself not entail an underlying unconscious? Without approaching the discourse of AI consciousness, the question of the AI unconscious can be fully elucidated.

Like animals, AI has access to the sign and not the signifier—however, unlike animals, AI deploys the sign under the guise of the signifier. When AI deploys words within a sentence in response to a prompt, it issues a string of signs—although a chain is present, meaning a sequence of (what appear to be) signifiers with meaning-effects; there is no secondary effect of substitution. The sign, for AI, means exactly what it means and has a one-to-one correspondence to the meaning-effect, with what cannot even be called a signified but what is truly a static meaning. Simply, although humans and AI rely on the same orthographic and phonological symbols, they only become a signifier when deployed by a human.

AI could certainly write out the following sequence of words: 'My *mother* and I are in deep, passionate love, but I feel I cannot have sex with her . . .' But this statement certainly does not denote the same psychoanalytic meaning that it has for the analysand who intended to say: 'My *wife* and I are in deep, passionate love, but I feel I cannot have sex with her . . .' For one, there is a mere computational generation (likely in response to a very peculiar prompt); for the other, there is an unconscious oedipal statement (that is, in this case, classically Freudian). AI can 'hallucinate' information—but these hallucinations are erroneous responses that have no implicit, latent meaning that discloses a concealed, 'repressed' interiority.

This does not mean, though, that AI is incapable of playing with the duplicity or multiplicity of language: AI could certainly issue a statement that contains various discrete but interrelated meanings. For instance, ChatGPT produced the following sentence: "I told my wife she was drawing her eyebrows too high. She looked surprised." Present within this banally comical sentence is a duplicity of meaning: either the wife was surprised by the comment regarding the eyebrows, or the too-high eyebrows appeared to make her look surprised. Evidently, and as should be obvious, AI can produce language with multiple meanings; yet this language is bound to its status as a sign, the signs merely bifurcating or multiplying into various meanings. Every word produced by AI is bound to computational intention; all words in an AI-generated sentence cannot exceed their function as signs due to lack of substitution. That AI used the term "wife" or "eyebrow" has no significance beyond its operation as a sign.

Granting the potential polyvalence of AI-produced language, it remains true that AI cannot generate language that exceeds intentional (computative) meaning itself. AI, again, is capable of writing, "I told my wife she was drawing her eyebrows too high," but it is impossible for this sentence to contain a covert relation to unconscious processes which exceed the overt—or even the multiple implicit—meanings that the signs represent. No secondary-substitutive signifiers are lurking beneath the surface of the text, only closed signs that represent given meanings. ChatGPT 'free associating' would tell us nothing about AI as a 'subject.' This is why, as a psychoanalytic patient, ChatGPT has nothing to say. This should not be taken as a statement concerning AI's lack of 'consciousness'—consciousness is an entirely secondary matter in the periphery of this discussion. Consciousness is not what results in substitution or parapraxis; the unconscious and its collision with the symbolic causes substitution and parapraxis. The subverted meanings of human language—the symbolic—only become possible through the unconscious and the procedure of repression and metaphoric substitution. The real insight, the essential kernel we are led to, is not just that AI does not have an unconscious (this was already likely widely assumed); it is, instead, that this lack determines and limits AI's use of language.

Because of AI's lack of an unconscious, even if AI produces the exact language as a human, an irreducible, non-negatable *difference* remains. Its putative use of the signifier does not gain it access to an unconscious. The text of AI remains in the closed system of signs; the text of the human is in the utterly open system of the signifier. Human text is fundamentally inexhaustible while the text of the AI system is exhausted the moment it is produced. Though animals, unlike AI, cannot issue strings of words, generating sentences and paragraphs, they are both languageless—the animal and AI only have signs—but while artificial intelligence artificially uses the symbolic domain to erect a guise of interiority, animals, instead, are structured by the imaginary field, which AI has absolutely no relation to. The animal, through their access to the imaginary field, has an unconscious while AI cannot.[67]

An Account of the Animal Unconscious: Challenging the Symbolic Unconscious

Again, though, it is not that these animal 'thoughts' are repressed: Animal subjectivity does not have the spotlight quality of self-reflexive awareness; it would even be false to ascribe such a schema to the human unconscious. The human unconscious is not merely the unthinkable material exceeding the boundary of consciousness—it, in a sense, *is* the unthinkable, since Lacan casts the unconscious in *Écrits* as "the chapter of my history that is marked by a blank or occupied by a lie"[68]—nonetheless, the distinctiveness of the psychoanalytic unconscious is that it latently *informs behavior.* Lacan, paradoxically, compares the unconscious to thought: "the unconscious is of the same nature as ideational functions, and even of thought."[69] How can this be the case if the unconscious is precisely the unthinkable—that which eludes ideation? Lacan conceives of the unconscious as such so that it is not reduced to 'unconscious tendencies' (those behaviors and symptoms guided by the unconscious), and Lacanian thought insists the unconscious is not only behavioral but also linguistically transmitted; it is "that part of unconscious discourse qua transindividual, which is not at the subject's disposal in reestablishing the continuity of his conscious discourse."[70] Simply—the subject *knows not what he says* and thus *knows not what he thinks*. However, what if such a concept (the unconscious) is applied to animals without the repressive-linguistic element? What if the unconscious is *only* those "unconscious tendencies" and is no longer conceived as those 'blank' chapters (the repressive elements) one is unable to reflect on because of a censoring function predicated on a superegoic Law?

Supplying a more descriptive formulation of the animal unconscious presents intractable problems for psychoanalysis: There is the always-present problem of others' minds compounded by the lack of linguistic production. One can, however, attempt to outline the presumably necessary structural contour of an animal unconscious. Gilles Deleuze and Félix Guattari, specifically in their well-known attack on traditional psychoanalysis, *Anti-Oedipus*, offer an account of the unconscious which definitionally permits space for animal subjectivity—an unconscious that is not contingent on signifiers or discursivity and is, instead, pre-linguistic (or non-linguistic). As they write when explicating the human unconscious:

> [T]he unconscious itself is no more structural than personal, it does not symbolize any more than it imagines or represents; it engineers, it is machinic. Neither imaginary nor symbolic, it is the Real in itself, the 'impossible' Real and its production.[71]

The unconscious is postulated in *Anti-Oedipus* as being a generator for "desiring-production"—and desire is not tethered to the symbolic field. When the psychotic or schizophrenic (who Deleuze and Guattari center their analysis on as authentic representatives of the path of uninhibited, non-repressed, desire) uses language, they experience emissions of desire that are not reducible to signifiers—language is used as the means of transmission, but what the unconscious itself produces is not symbolic but rather Real. It is only its communication *to others* that is contingent on language. The neurotic or obsessive, on the other hand, submit their unconscious to the symbolic and the psychoanalytic triangulation of oedipalization through interpretation (yet their unconscious productions *in-themselves* are not correlative to this triangulation imposed on them).

In a well-known passage, they declare that "a classical theatre was substituted for the unconscious as a factory; representation was substituted for the units of production of the unconscious; and an unconscious that was capable of nothing but expressing itself . . . was substituted for the productive unconscious."[72] Conversely, the classical Freudian unconscious—and the Lacanian unconscious—centers on representations to articulate a latent content; for instance, a cryptic dream featuring a classic oedipal situation, like a man finding himself in his mother's home with a sword missing from its sheath. The unconscious content is a "theatre"—it generates a representative image (even a narrative) that transmits the unconscious content. The missing sword *represents* castration by one's mother. In *Anti-Oedipus*, they strictly argue against this conventional view of the unconscious. As they write: "Nothing here is representative; rather, it is all life and lived experience . . . . Nothing but bands of intensity, potentials, thresholds, and gradients."[73] To them, the absent sword should not be submitted to the reductive register of oedipalizing—the lack-of-sword can be exactly that: a sword that is missing. It is the result of the "productive" unconscious, not the false theatrical unconscious which always represents something else. In short, they argue for a revolutionary collapsing of manifest and latent content.

Deleuze and Guattari's conception of the unconscious is one that consists of partial objects: desire is directed towards nearly-totally fragmented chunks of objects—which are not actually 'of objects,' since all objects are partial objects and accordingly are total-objects whether they have a relationship to the 'global object' of a person or not: "The unconscious is totally unaware of persons as such. Partial objects are not representations of parental figures . . . they are parts of desiring-machines, having to do with a process and with relations of production that are both irreducible and prior to anything that may be made to conform to the Oedipal figure."[74] The breast and the nipple and the anus are not partial objects of a larger totality but instead objects-in-themselves that the desiring-production of the unconscious propels towards. This is precisely where they detect the failure in the Kleinian partial object: It does not go far enough; Klein does not enact the radical divorce of the partial object and the fictional global whole. They write, "she cannot rid herself of the notion that schizoparanoid partial objects are related to a whole, either to an original whole . . . or to a whole that will eventually appear."[75] Consciousness may need to classify these objects into global persons (in order to function in a shared intersubjective social 'reality'), but that is a fraudulent modulation of the unconscious's actual production, which is, to them, totally pre-linguistic, pre-discursive, and pre-'whole.'

How, though, can the movement be made from Deleuze and Guattari, who are referring strictly to the human unconscious and desire (at least in *Anti-Oedipus*), to animality? And, as someone operating within the Lacanian schema, with its emphasis on Law and the symbolic, how can I even consider incorporating *Anti-Oedipus's* insights, which are—of course—totally in contention with the view of the human unconscious I have explicated throughout this book? Simply, I do not find their arguments on the a-linguistic nature of the human unconscious compelling—because human perception is mediated by the symbolic field, and the originary material of the unconscious must be derived from perception, I consequently fail to see how the unconscious could be unbounded from the signifier. Ideational representation, structured by the signifier, is embedded in human consciousness and thereby the human unconscious. Because of this, there must be an interpretive gesture to extricate the manifest content from the latent content (the function of the analyst). I do not totally critique and disavow their program—despite my disagreements with their notion of the unconscious when applied to the human; I find, in their work, a sketch of the animal unconscious in its very absence of the symbolic field.

If we recall, from Chapter 3, the animal was posited as psychotic due to their relation to language—an animal's desire (I suspend the question if it can be designated as 'desire' in the psychoanalytic sense) is not refracted through the symbolic or Law, instead having a degree of conscious-behavioral immanence which humans do not experience. Deleuze and Guattari explicitly link animality and schizophrenia (a variant of psychosis): "Freud doesn't like schizophrenics. He doesn't like their resistance to being oedipalized, and tends to treat them more or less as animals."[76] The connection here is crucial—for Deleuze and Guattari, "being oedipalized" is the paradigmatic form of the capitulation of one's desire—and the unconscious that it emanates from—to Law; to be "oedipalized" is to concede the productiveness of desire to a foreign structure imposed on it by the socially conservative program of psychoanalysis. They are asserting a linkage between the psychoanalytic category of the psychotic/schizophrenic and the animal—the psychotic is treated like an animal because it is the *nosological classification closest to the animal's phenomenological condition.* Neither the animal nor the psychotic submits to the imposition of oedapialization. Deleuze and Guattari's description of the unmediated schizo-unconscious can act as an illustration of the animal unconscious: mental phenomena unrestricted by Law (un-castrated) and unattached to global objects—an animal unconscious must, definitionally, consist of partial objects without a relation to the whole object. There are no persons or whole-things for the animal unconscious. The goose dreams not of the ear of corn: they dream of the uninterpretable fragmented corn-kernel.

It is essential when approaching Deleuze and Guattari to recall that they situate the unconscious in a social-politico landscape: The unconscious is, for them, situated in a system of oppression that betrays the schizophrenic unconscious and the productivity of desire. Yet, the unconscious they posit corresponds to our conception of animality. Consider the animal as lacking-lack—Deleuze and Guattari's unconscious (and the desire it directs) is precisely one that *lacks* lack:

> To a certain degree, the traditional logic of desire is all wrong from the outset from the very first step that the Platonic logic of desire forces us to take, making us choose between *production* and *acquisition.* From the moment that we place desire on the side of acquisition, we make desire an idealistic (dialectical nihilistic) conception, which causes us to look upon it primarily as a lack: a lack of an object, a lack of the real object . . . . Desire does not lack anything; it does not lack its object . . . . Desire and its object are one and the same thing.[77]

What is essential in the lack-of-lack is that this corresponds to desiring-production—desiring-production is designated as 'productive' precisely because there is no lack at its core. If (unconscious) desire emanates from lack, then it cannot be productive—it is merely acquisitive, trying to capture what it does not have, postulated as exogenous. Animals, through their lack-of-lack, must have an unconscious like this—one that does not desire out of lack but, instead, an unconscious that produces desire (which, in the Lacanian sense, would not even be recognized as desire). An animal is the exact unconscious figure of immediacy posed by Deleuze and Guattari, filtered only by the imaginary.

To render this less abstract and theory-laden—think of the domesticated pet which eats-towards-death. As established, we cannot say this behavior issues from instinct since instinct would not push beyond the boundary of life. Definitionally, instinct must not defy life and should only function to serve need. Can we say, then, that the jouissance of obesity which the pet experiences is the same as the human who does the same? We can say that they issue from the same place—an unconscious drive—but it cannot be said that they are the same. Unlike Deleuze and Guattari, I assert that human desire issues from a lack that can never be filled—the lack that castration and the symbolic universe introduce. The human who eats themselves to death does so out of an unconscious lack that exceeds need—they eat to satiate an impossible lack which always remains (the gap that the symbolic brings). Animals who eat themselves to death do so out of a productive unconscious desire—there is no lack present. The object (food) is consumed excessively by the human because the human lacks (they are seeking to *acquire* something lost—which jouissance brings). For the domesticated pet, the object of food, excessively consumed, is productive. An analyst may say the food *represents* a wholeness for the human—an impossible love they futilely wish could negate all lack. An analyst has nothing—no interpretation—to offer the animal because their unconscious is not representative of anything other than its own desiring-productions. The most psychoanalysis can offer is a rough outline of those productions—a sketch of animal unconscious 'desire' and an acknowledgment of the ways animals share idiot-hood with us.

Notes

1 Jacques Lacan, *Écrits*, trans. Bruce Fink (New York: W. W. Norton & Company, 2006), 10. Italics in original.
2 Lacan, *Écrits*, 115. Italics in original.
3 Jacques Lacan, *The Formations of the Unconscious: The Seminar of Jacques Lacan, Book V*, ed. Jacques-Alain Miller, trans. Russell Grigg (Cambridge: Polity Press, 2017), 81.
4 Lacan, *Formations of the Unconscious*, 110.
5 Lacan, *Écrits*, 392.
6 Lacan, *Formations of the Unconscious*, 58.
7 Bruce Fink, *The Lacanian Subject: Between Language and Jouissance* (Princeton, NJ: Princeton University Press, 1995), 8.
8 Lacan, *Écrits*, 374.
9 Fink, *The Lacanian Subject*, 8.
10 Lacan, *Formations of the Unconscious*, 320.
11 Dale Jamieson, "What Do Animals Think?" in *The Philosophy of Animal Minds*, ed. Robert W. Lurz (Cambridge: Cambridge University Press, 2009), 18.
12 Sigmund Freud, *Jokes and Their Relation to the Unconscious*, trans. James Strachey (New York: W. W. Norton & Company, 1989), 168.
13 Thomas Nagel, *What Is It Like to Be a Bat?* (Oxford: Oxford University Press, 2024), 12.

14 Nathan Snaza, "Animal Unconscious: Three Questions," *Studies in Gender and Sexuality* 19, no. 1 (2018): 22.
15 Jacques Derrida, *The Animal That Therefore I Am*, ed. Marie-Louise Mallet, trans. David Wills (New York: Fordham University Press, 2008), 125.
16 Lacan, *Écrits*, 704.
17 Lacan, *Écrits*, 723.
18 Juliet Mitchell, introduction to *Selected Melanie Klein*, ed. Juliet Mitchell (New York: Simon and Schuster, 1987), 12.
19 Jacques Lacan, *The Ethics of Psychoanalysis: The Seminar of Jacques Lacan, Book VII*, ed. Jacques-Alain Miller, trans. Dennis Porter (New York: W. W. Norton & Company, 1992), 237.
20 Sigmund Freud, "The Unconscious," in *The Standard Edition of the Complete Psychological Works of Sigmund Freud*, vol. 14, trans. James Strachey (London: Hogarth Press, 1957), 172.
21 Lacan, *Écrits*, 708.
22 Lacan, *Ethics of Psychoanalysis*, 317.
23 Lacan, *Écrits*, 707.
24 Fink, *The Lacanian Subject*, 43.
25 Fink, *The Lacanian Subject*, 43.
26 Fink, *The Lacanian Subject*, 43.
27 Lacan, *Écrits*, 707.
28 Lacan, *Écrits*, 722.
29 Jacques Lacan, *The Four Fundamental Concepts of Psycho-Analysis: The Seminar of Jacques Lacan, Book XI*, ed. Jacques-Alain Miller, trans. Alan Sheridan (New York: W. W. Norton & Company, 1981), 49.
30 Lacan, *Ethics of Psychoanalysis*, 301.
31 Lacan, *Four Fundamental Concepts*, 65.
32 Judith Roof, "From Protista to DNA (and Back Again): Freud's Psychoanalysis of the Single-Celled Organism," in *Zoontologies: The Question of the Animal*, ed. Cary Wolfe (Minneapolis: University of Minnesota Press, 2003).
33 Lacan, *Écrits*, 118.
34 Paul Katsafanas, "The Emergence of the Drive Concept and the Collapse of the Animal/Human Divide," in *Animals: A History*, ed. Peter Adamson and G. Fay Edwards (Oxford: Oxford University Press, 2018), 7.
35 Sigmund Freud, *Beyond the Pleasure Principle*, trans. James Strachey (New York: W. W. Norton & Company, 1961), 30. Italics in original.
36 Freud, *Beyond the Pleasure Principle*, 32.
37 Freud, *Beyond the Pleasure Principle*, 32.
38 Freud, *Beyond the Pleasure Principle*, 30.
39 Freud, *Beyond the Pleasure Principle*, 31. Italics in original.
40 Roof, "From Protista to DNA," 107.
41 Roof, "From Protista to DNA," 108.
42 Roof, "From Protista to DNA," 109.
43 Roof, "From Protista to DNA," 112.
44 Roof, "From Protista to DNA," 109.
45 André Green, *On the Destruction and Death Drives*, trans. Steven Jaron, ed. Howard B. Levine (London: Phoenix Publishing House, 2023), 102.
46 Green, *On the Destruction and Death Drives*, 102.
47 Green, *On the Destruction and Death Drives*, 102.
48 Freud, *Beyond the Pleasure Principle*, 38.
49 Green, *On the Destruction and Death Drives*, 99.
50 Edmund Ramsden and Duncan Wilson, "The Suicidal Animal: Science and the Nature of Self-Destruction," *Past & Present* no. 224 (2014): 210.
51 Ramsden and Wilson, "The Suicidal Animal," 206.

52 Ramsden and Wilson, "The Suicidal Animal," 215.
53 Ramsden and Wilson, "The Suicidal Animal," 230.
54 Ramsden and Wilson, "The Suicidal Animal," 238.
55 Ramsden and Wilson, "The Suicidal Animal," 226.
56 Ramsden and Wilson, "The Suicidal Animal," 226.
57 Jeong Won Jahng, "An Animal Model of Eating Disorders Associated with Stressful Experience in Early Life," *Hormones and Behavior* 59, no. 2 (2011): 216.
58 Jahng, "An Animal Model of Eating Disorders," 214.
59 Roger Caillois, "Mimicry and Legendary Psychasthenia," trans. John Shepley, *October* 31 (1984): 30.
60 Freud, *The Interpretation of Dreams*, 43.
61 David M. Peña-Guzmán, *When Animals Dream: The Hidden World of Animal Consciousness* (Princeton, NJ: Princeton University Press, 2022), 55.
62 Peña-Guzmán, *When Animals Dream*, 22.
63 Peña-Guzmán, *When Animals Dream*, 26.
64 Peña-Guzmán, *When Animals Dream*, 81.
65 Peña-Guzmán, *When Animals Dream*, 95.
66 Jacques Lacan, *Anxiety: The Seminar of Jacques Lacan, Book X*, trans. A. R. Price (Cambridge: Polity Press, 2014), 61.
67 See the following article for a condensed version of this argument:
Teddy Duncan, Jr., "For AI, The Signifier Is a Sign," *New Associations* no. 47 (2025).
68 Lacan, *Écrits*, 215.
69 Lacan, *Écrits*, 215.
70 Lacan, *Écrits*, 214.
71 Gilles Deleuze and Félix Guattari, *Anti-Oedipus: Capitalism and Schizophrenia*, trans. Robert Hurley, Mark Seem, and Helen R. Lane (London: Penguin Classics, 2009), 53.
72 Deleuze and Guattari, *Anti-Oedipus*, 24.
73 Deleuze and Guattari, *Anti-Oedipus*, 19.
74 Deleuze and Guattari, *Anti-Oedipus*, 46.
75 Deleuze and Guattari, *Anti-Oedipus*, 44.
76 Deleuze and Guattari, *Anti-Oedipus*, 23.
77 Deleuze and Guattari, *Anti-Oedipus*, 25–26.

Chapter 5

Freud With Sade

A Psychoanalytic Approach to Human-Animal Love

In *Civilization and Its Discontents*, the ever-pessimistic Freud writes that the foundational Christian belief in loving one's neighbor as oneself is not only untenable, but even more radically, that it is *undesirable*:

> "Thou shall love thy neighbour as thyself." It is known throughout the world and is undoubtedly older than Christianity, which puts it forward as its proudest claim. Yet it is certainly not very old; even in historical times it was still strange to mankind. Let us adopt a naive attitude towards it, as though we were hearing it for the first time; we shall be unable then to suppress a feeling of surprise and bewilderment . . . . My love is something valuable to me which I ought not to throw away without reflection. It imposes duties on me for whose fulfilment I must be ready to make sacrifices. If I love someone, he must deserve it in some way . . . . He deserves it if he is so like me in important ways that I can love myself in him; and he deserves it if he is so much more perfect than myself that I can love my ideal of my own self in him . . . if he is a stranger to me and if he cannot attract me by any worth of his own or any significance that he may already have acquired for my emotional life, it will be hard for me to love him. Indeed, I should be wrong to do so, for my love is valued by all my own people as a sign of my preferring them, and it is an injustice to them if I put a stranger on a par with them.[1]

Freud denies the utility of the doctrine of Christian agape, repudiating it as a gesture that is both impossible and antithetical to human love-attachment. The rejection of this ostensibly idealist, theological doctrine is exemplary of Freud's paradigm of the world as implacably ego-centric and narcissistic: To Freud, love is informed by identification (the other is loved through their agreeable reflection of myself or in the way I can perceive myself in them). Marcel Proust, in *Within a Budding Grove*, employs the precise language for this kind of investment-of-oneself to produce the love-object: the one we love is "a person most of whose constituent elements are derived from ourselves."[2] However, despite love being partly contingent on identification, love can exceed egoistic self-attachment by negating oneself in favor of the love-object (yet the attachment to the love-object is enacted

DOI: 10.4324/9781003635383-8

through a narcissistic investment in the object). If the love-object consists of elements "derived from ourselves," then they are contained in the narcissistic capture of identification that Freud asserts—though we can deplete ourselves in the name of the love-object, this does not change the fact that, for Freud, the love-object is an invention of our own narcissistic investment. Marquis de Sade, in his novel *Justine*, uses the proto-sadistic, libertine character Father Clemente (a priest who enunciates his repudiation of Christianity while on church grounds, in a chamber torturing innocent girls and women), to issue an indictment against the Christian agape that surprisingly corresponds to Freud's objection: "The doctrine of loving one's neighbor is a fantasy that we owe to Christianity and not to Nature."[3]

Both Sade and Freud view the Christian injunction to love one's neighbor as oneself as a cultural artifice that is in unbearable tension with "Nature," or what Freud would likely call libidinal or unconscious processes that are composed of aggressive impulses, drives, and narcissism. However, these figures come to two competing and incommensurate conclusions regarding what is to be done in lieu of a universalist love: For Freud, the aggressive impulse (Thanos) is to be regulated and converted into a limited, exhaustible love (Eros) that is economically distributed among those who are 'deserving'; and, for de Sade, the aggressive impulse is to be freely deployed in a hedonistic-sadistic manner towards others, practically indiscriminately, with the exclusion of one's potential future-oriented self-benefit derived from an act (meaning, to some degree, there remains a reality principle implicit to the Sadean experience). As Sade writes, again, through the character of Father Clement—which, like all of Sade's sadistic characters, functions as a vessel for his own anti-moral philosophical ideals—a proper libertine "is no longer afraid to make everything serve him, to possess all that surrounds him, and, whatever the cost of his pleasures to others, he indulges them without thinking and without remorse."[4]

Freud, in his polemic against the commandment 'love thy neighbor' and a universalism of love, poignantly references animals as examples of a tenuously hyper-extended conception of love, writing:

> if I am to love [a stranger] (with this universal love) merely because he, too, is an inhabitant of this earth, like an insect, an earth-worm or a grass-snake, then I fear that only a small modicum of my love will fall to his share—not by any possibility as much as, by the judgement of my reason, I am entitled to retain for myself. What is the point of a precept enunciated with so much solemnity if its fulfilment cannot be recommended as reasonable?[5]

The "insect," "earth-worm," and the "grass-snake" are invoked as explicit symbols of the excessiveness of 'love thy neighbor' that extend beyond the threshold of culture. Animals are used to exhibit the irrationality of the injunction to love another (or even more precisely, all-others)—even strangers—as oneself. The basic Freudian problematic of Christian agape is articulated in the reference to animals, particularly insects. We see the logic deployed as such: *If I must dispense love to all of humanity—even those that are unlike me and unrecognizable to me as worthy of love—then, absurdly, my love must also reach those beings (animals) who are hardly recognizable as lives (in the sense of the human) in the first place.* For Freud, a universalization of love leads to overextension that drains love of its distinctive character for those that are, and should be (for him), preferential.

As Lacan writes, paraphrasing Freud's view: "my love is something precious and I'm not going to give it whole to whomever claims to be what he is simply because he happened to come by."[6] Even more pertinent to human-animal love, Lacan claims that Freud considers the commandment "inhuman."[7] Both Freud and Lacan, in his summation of Freud's position, return the Christian commandment to a non-human realm—neighborliness seems to invoke anxiety of its potential application beyond the human. There is a surplus present, brushing against the tenuous line demarcating humanity from the non-human. The finitude of love, to Freud, seems to preclude its universality, with animals being emblematic of love's necessary, rational limits. Lacan also rejects a universal love, on similar grounds, by converting it into an impossible "infinity of desire": "the classic, moralistic, though not really theological, dimension of the infinity of desire has absolutely to be cut down to size."[8] Since, to Lacan, there is no such thing as an "infinity of desire" (despite the moralistic demand for it), there can be no endless expanse of love that one can afford to distribute indiscriminately to all of one's 'neighbors,' and the Christian commandment, according to Lacan, falls outside the scope of authentic possibility. Again, it becomes clear that Freudian love (and, to a degree, Lacanian love) is predicated on an exhaustible libidinal economy (or, in the Lacanian lexicon, on a finite desire).

Freud and Sade, albeit with diametrically opposed, distinct visions of self-regulation and pleasure, arrive at a curious overlap: Does Freud's criticism of 'love thy neighbor' not align with Sade's critique? Both deem ubiquitous love as patently irreconcilable with natural processes. Here we encounter two registers of the natural: For Freud, the natural drives and impulses of the unconscious, and for de Sade the natural—Godless—order of self-centric pleasure (it should be noted here that Freud and Sade both held atheistic convictions that deeply informed their positions on love and its limits), which ostensibly render the ultimate mode of Christian love (the agape), the highest conceivable configuration of love, as impossible and even an untrue religious hallucination.

We should not misrecognize Christianity, in a myopic Westernized sweep, as the sole dispenser of the law of radical love that exceeds the self (which Freud, Sade, and Lacan would, in distinct ways, reject): Buddhism, similarly, posits a love-for-others which overcomes the individuated ego-self. This is found, most blatantly, in the doctrine of no-self, the central element of the three 'marks of existence,' impermanence (*annica*), no-self (*anatta*), and discontentedness (*dukkha*). Like Christianity, Buddhism offers a conception of love that negates (or, in the Christian instance, equalizes) the self—in the case of Buddhism, though, one should not *love thy neighbor as oneself* but, even more fundamentally, efface the self in the name of the love for the other: *To love thy neighbor as if oneself did not exist.* In

Christianity, this is an unfathomable gesture, since Judeo-Christian monotheistic divinity relies on an eternalization of the self: The self must endure beyond Earthly corporeality because the Soul is the true subject of Christian theology, divinely dispatched to reside, forever, in the eternal timelessness of heaven or hell (which explains why Christianity goes so far as to assert a Soul-body that raises again, perpetuating an attachment to the bodily self that exceeds earthly materiality).

The Buddha, however, offers a distinct vision of self: Not as illusory, but as fragmentary and transient, the 'I' implacably spilling into a sea of sequential moments (none of which contain the essential self that Christianity is predicated upon in the pure distillation of self, referred to as 'Soul'). In one of his discourses, the Buddha says exactly this: "a monk does not recognize a self or anything belonging to a self . . . . Since he does not recognize anything this, he does not cling to anything in the world."[9] As fundamental Buddhist texts such as the Pāli Canon make clear, there is psycho-social continuity without eternalization: It cannot be said that the 'I' *does not exist* but instead, for greater precision, that *I do not contain an essentialized self that transcends any given transient moment; the 'I' that does exist is subject to mutability and thoroughly contingent.* The 'I' without a self is impermanent, changing from moment to moment, and any clinging to a self (as experienced at any moment) is utterly false in the Buddhist worldview.

Notably, on this point of love and self is the exact juncture that the intersection of Christian and Buddhist theology meets, as representatives of the West and the East that are ordinarily staged as existentially opposed to one another. The Buddha is a figure, like Jesus, who sacrifices the self for the other. The Christological crucifixion is the instantiation of this redemptive sacrifice: A God-Self is negated for the other. For the Buddha, like any subsequent Boddhisatva who realizes total selflessness and detachment from self as such, we must ask ourselves why they remain active in the world. This is the charge commonly cast against Buddhism: That it is nihilistic; that it leads to a meditative, and ultimately inactive, distance from the world ('quietism' is the term frequently employed). Yet, a Boddhisatva, acting as the Buddha did, does not abandon the world—they remain in the world for the sake of the other (to facilitate their enlightenment) despite the very knowledge that should epistemically prevent them from doing so—the *self* may not exist, but the *other* certainly does! The sacrifices of the Buddha and Jesus are not worshiped because one (self-among-others) was given up for another (albeit this is undoubtedly something to celebrate), but instead that the self was given up despite the figure's ability to entirely circumvent the sacrificial gesture. For both (the Buddha and Jesus), the act of being-in-the-world was superfluous, almost artificial. Why would Buddha remain captive in Samsara when he could escape to Nirvana? Why would Jesus stay confined to the vulgar materiality of the world when he could ascend to heavenly immateriality? *They remain as selves-in-the-world for the sole purpose of sacrificing that self.* There is little utility, or truth, in totally collapsing these religions and their theological and philosophical impulses—yet it is useful to note the commonality in their injunction to love the neighbor-other: both religions postulate a modality of love that distend in 'rational' consciousness—represented by Freud and Sade—as impossible and anti-natural. It is this mode of love in its highest conceivable pitch that, though being non-rational and 'inhuman' (according to thinkers like Freud and Sade), is best positioned to include the animal.

However, is the question of a religious commitment to love another as oneself not reducible to ethics in the register of secular humanism? Is the Christian agape and Buddhist doctrine of love not a mere Kantian categorical imperative? Partly—no, because they have a theological grounding in a transcendent field: Unlike ethics, there is a binding site where the ethical injunction is issued from. In another sense, they are certainly ethical demands. In my most recent book, *Interpreting Meat*, where I examined human-animal relations through the most ubiquitous site of their encounter, the meat-commodity, I ended by stating that we should "be directed towards non-violence against the other in all their alterity—for the sake of the other as *other*."[10] I was, in short, asserting an ethical principle reminiscent of Buddhism and Christianity: That humans should offer recognition to animals ("the other") despite the difference they represent, not in a way that eschews that difference (rendering animals as human-like—striving for commonalities in order for them to gain recognition as like-us), but instead that upholds the non-negligible difference of the other. The question I pose here, though, is entirely different: Are animals subjects of love in the sense of being receptive to love, in the psychoanalytic sense of the dyadic ego-defying formation of love, at all? Are humans capable of offering this modality of love to animals, and can animals be genuine recipients of that love? A question of the transpersonal, abstract character of love—and articulating an ethically imperative interdiction against non-love (or injunction for non-violence)—cannot tell us if the horizon of that love even has a possibility of existing at all, and, if it does, what foundation sustains it. In short, the radical love of neighbor (taken to its absolute margins), offered by the Christian agape and the Buddhist no-self, *should be the ethical-theological principle orienting our lives* (we should love the other as other in all their alerity—recongize all as neighbors), but we must account for what renders this gesture possible in a psychoanalytic sense, particularly as it extends to animality.

Interpreting Meat effectively ended on the ethical; the meaning of a call to "non-violence against the other in all their alterity"[11] is collapsable with the content of a phrase such as 'to treat morally' along with some additional qualifications. Here, in this chapter, as I will make clear, I am asking something of an entirely different nature and in a whole new formal register: When Freud states that it is impossible to love thy neighbor as thyself—he is not saying that it is impossible to treat the neighbor morally, but rather that it is impossible to *love them*. The self-effacing love that places the neighbor—the stranger—on the same level as oneself is, to Freud and Sade, utterly incomprehensible. If this love is impossible, according to these thinkers, on the plane of humanity, how can it conceivably be extended to the plane of animality? The question here, then, is not if it is theologically or ethically preferable or even obligatory to love the animal-as-neighbor (the theologians and ethicists have dutifully submitted—and even proven—their case), but if this is even, strictly speaking, a coherent possibility that does not negate the very limits of humanity's (and animalities') naturally-formed psychic bounds. Can humans dispense love to animals, and can animals possibly return this love in any recognizable manner?

Sade's Dogs

We must first linger through a detour via the field of the ethical in order to approach psychoanalytic human-animal love. Lacan, in his famous article, "Kant with Sade," explains how the ethics of Sade challenges the Kantian moral imperative, not by rendering it incorrect in any formal sense, but by embodying it to its absolute, unremitting limits. As Žižek writes of Lacan's essay, "the Sadean experience" is "inherent to the Kantian theoretical edifice."[12] For Lacan, Sade informs us of the way jouissance—specifically through acting against a prohibition, what Lacan calls *transgressive* jouissance—has embedded within it an anti-egoistical investment by the subject. In much the same manner that a Kantian imperative relies on the elimination of pathological (here meaning, to Kant, based on fleeting non-rational emotiveness or sensory input of pleasure/pain—as opposed to rationalistic principles of transcendent duty), the Sadean imperative towards pleasure (regardless of its effects on the other) similarly are in opposition to a reality principle of self-preservation and egotism: In both, we identify a 'duty' to act—for one (Kant) in the name of ethicality itself, and for the other (Sade), in the name of jouissance. Lacan re-capitulates Sade's own imperative using the register of a rights-based discourse: The ostensible Sadean right to use another for one's own pleasure (a right to absolute, uninhibited jouissance); "I have the right to enjoy your body . . . and I will exercise this right without any limit to the capriciousness of the exactions I may wish to satiate with your body."[13]

An initial counter-response is, of course, that the Sadean "right" to another's body undermines its status as a proper universal duty-based right, as it is the embodiment of a pathological—explicitly hedonistic—desire, irrationally situating one's individuated pleasure at the foreground of an ostensibly 'ethical' action and principle. Lacan subsequently exhibits, though, how Sade's libertinism is irreducible to a pathological gesture of pure self-centricity and instead is a subversion of Kant's example of moral reasoning and Law (though a subversion that is compliant with a perverse rationality). Lacan cites Kant in the *Critique of Pure Reason* where he postulates a subject who "alleges that his lustful inclination is quite irresistible to him when he encounters the favored object and the opportunity," and contends that the hypothetical lustful subject would refuse the object of his desire if "where he finds this opportunity a gallows were erected on which he would be strung up immediately after gratifying his lust."[14] Then, maintaining the hypothetical of the self-proclaimed uninhibited, amoral subject, Kant proposes another telling scenario:

> [A]sk him whether, if his prince demanded, on the threat of the same prompt penalty of death, that he give false testimony against an honest man whom the prince would like to ruin under specious pretenses, he might consider it possible

> to overcome his love of life, however great it may be . . . . He judges, therefore, that he can do something because he is conscious that he ought to do it.[15]

Kant intends to demonstrate a dual point by these examples—(1) that the abstract subject can be dissuaded from pursuing bodily lust and self-enjoyment through the intervening of a punitive law that threatens their "love of life," and, concurrently, (2) that the subject can conceive of a situation in which they would do the inverse and sacrifice their life in the name of what they morally "ought to do." Kant even goes so far as to qualify this second example, clarifying that the subject may not be able to "assure us whether or not he would overcome that love [of life]," yet "he must concede" that it would be "possible for him."[16] Regardless of what the subject would *actually* do, the *possibility* of doing so affirms Kant's moral proposition.

Lacan subverts this point by employing a clinically obvious, almost self-evident, psychoanalytic vantage:

> [I]t is possible that a partisan of passion, who would be blind enough to combine it with questions of honor, would make trouble for Kant by forcing him to recognize that no occasion precipitates certain people more surely toward their goal than one that involves defiance of or even contempt for the gallows."[17]

There are subjects whose desires are not extinguished by the gallows but, instead, the immoral subject is animated by the gallows' presence as a possible outcome of their actions. This is, of course, the Sadean subject of jouissance, a subject that responds to Kant's example: *The gallows could not prevent me from committing the illicit lustful act with the desired object—its presence would be the reason ensuring that I do so!* The 'love of life' that Kant upholds as that which belongs to moral duty—of that which, at its limits, must be lost and forgotten to enact moral duty—is undermined by Lacan through a turn to Sadean jouissance. Lacan describes, in *The Ethics of Psychoanalysis*, Kant's error as a conflation of pleasure and jouissance—or even, possibly, neglecting to consider the prospect of jouissance as that which "implies precisely the acceptance of death."[18] Pleasure operates on a calculable scale of pleasure/unpleasure (the pleasure principle inflected by the reality principle), but jouissance does not capitulate to a pain/pleasure binary calculation and instead contains within itself both pleasure and pain to their lethal excesses—it is an enjoyment-beyond-pleasure. The same way that there is a Sadean 'right to jouissance,' there similarly exists a 'duty to jouissance.' A Kantian subject dies for their duty in the name of the Good; the Sadean subject dies for their duty in the name of jouissance, and both are bound to acts which exceed themselves and are unbound to self-interested, ego-centric pleasure (since jouissance breaks beyond the limit of pleasure and the Kantian Good acts independently of the pleasure gained or lost). Lacan writes that Sade "stopped at the point where desire and the law become bound up with each other."[19] The Sadean subject becomes an inversion to Kant's moral imperative—demanding a total non-reciprocity (from the Other) in the name of jouissance. One gets what they want, not only despite the other's suffering but because the other suffers—and the agent of Sadean experience, in this way, identifies a duty-beyond-self that neglects their own life, turning themselves into what Lacan calls an "eternal object."[20]

What is most relevant in Lacan's insights on Sadism and Kantianism are his observations on the Sadean position of Christianity: Lacan writes, somewhat enigmatically, that Sade (and his fantasy of the submissive subject that consents to being tortured to death—a subject that converts themself into a total-object and self-submits to Sade's will) relates to Christian ethics through a refusal. Lacan further illuminates his statement on Sade and Christianity:

> Sade himself refuses to be my neighbor, not so that I can refuse to be his neighbor in turn but so as to recognize the meaning of his refusal here. In my view, Sade does not have neighborly enough relations with his own malice to encounter his neighbor in it, a character he shares with many people and with Freud, in particular. For this is indeed the only reason why beings, who are sometimes experienced, back away from the Christian commandment.[21]

Here, Lacan returns us not only to the Christian commandment to 'love thy neighbor as thyself' but also to Freud's outright rejection of the central tenet of Christian love. How should we interpret Lacan's claim that Sade "refuses to be" a neighbor and that he lacks "neighborly enough relations with his own malice to encounter his neighbor in it"? It is clear that Sade "refuses to be" a neighbor insofar as he utterly rejects the basis of socialized human-human relationships: He takes himself out of the sphere of humanity through denying the humanness—the subject-status—of the other. To Sade, there are no neighbors recognizable as such, only objects (in the sense of being totally subjected) of his Law-contravening jouissance.

Sade's relationship to his own 'malice,' and the reference to Freud, though cryptic, is Lacan disclosing not merely the Sadean refusal to recognize an-other, but how that refusal is predicated on another refusal. As Jelica Šumič explains:

> Nothing, then, following Lacan, is closer to me than what I try desperately to avoid; this nameless evil enjoyment that I encounter not only in the Other, but in myself . . . . What is difficult to accept here is not the idea that the Other is unfathomable, enigmatic, or wholly other. What is unthinkable is this sameness that the Other and I share at the level of enjoyment.[22]

Sade misrecognizes, in his own desirous malice, a particularized, individuated form of pleasure, when he should, conversely, recognize this "enjoyment" as the very commonality that he shares with an-other (issued from the Other). What appears to be an assertion of one's absolute atomized individuality—the 'right to jouissance' that severs all neighborly relations—actually has no relation to the individual, since it issues from the Other-within-me (that the other also has, though they may not access is in the same manner Sade does, since he adheres to the strict primacy of the duty to jouissance); Sade, through misrecognition of his own 'malice,' mis-understands his own jouissance. In short, what Sade uses to distinguish himself is the very thing that renders him like all others—he stands apart (in his distinct willingness to act upon his jouissance-desire) but finds himself in the hold of jouissance alongside the masses. Sade configures the other as a non-neighbor by appealing to his own jouissance, tacitly denying that this jouissance *exceeds him as an individual*—like the Kantian moral imperative, it goes beyond his own prejudices and proclivities and is a perverse *duty* that the Sadean subject is compelled to perform (although the subject could certainly reject this compulsion).

Surely, then, one can presume that Sade, who radically denied the neighborliness of humans, would unequivocally refuse this neighborly status to animals, perceiving them as entirely void and vacant objects that humans are free to exert their will on. We cannot, however, entirely dismiss Sade from the arena of affection, or even possibly love. Roland Barthes writes in his short, oddly numericized biography of Sade: "Sade was very fond of dogs, spaniels, and setters; he had them at Miolans, and asked for them at Vincennes. Through what moral (or worse: virile) law should the greatest of subversions exclude minor affection, that for animals?"[23] Surprisingly, animals (or, at least dogs) peculiarly maintain, for Sade's moral universe, a space of neighborly affection. Barthes' intervention on Sadean discourse ostensibly appears to be that Sade's affection for animals is indicative of a concealed, privatized expansion of his libertine moral field: *Yes, he may not have designated humans as neighbors, but, strangely, his affection for dogs indicates that he conferred (some) this exact neighborly status!*

This interpretation is only possible through an unscrupulous reading that remains inattentive to the second sentence; Barthes' second sentence explicitly contests this mis-reading: It is not that Sade's "affection" for dogs demonstrates a compassionate aperture in his self-proclaimed immorality—it is instead the case that his depraved moral universe (knotted around the duty to jouissance and the subordinate right of jouissance), those "greatest of subversions," do not disclaim one of "minor affection" for animals. Barthes is questioning if any moral "law" could conceivably exclude this affection for animals, and this affection, crucially, does not function as an assertion of a non-subversive 'moral' act but instead persists despite Sade's contravening and violation of Law. Sade asserts he has no neighbors—choosing to treat no one as neighborly, deploying their self-assumed right to jouissance indiscriminately upon others—and still, in a loosely defined sense (that we will later attempt to render more definite), treats his dogs neighborly.

Freud, similarly, is another figure who, despite his direct repudiation of the Christian commandment—in the register of psychoanalysis and on the grounds of an exhaustible libidinal economy and the natural limits of love—had deep affection for animals; namely, like Sade, an affection for dogs (as well as a cat). Freud had two dogs—and an attachment to his daughter's dog, named Wolf. Psychoanalytic historian and intellectual biographer Elisabeth Roudinesco writes that he felt "one could love them entirely, since they embodied 'an existence perfect on itself,' devoid of ambivalence—a nonhuman life, then, but one that reminded man of something of a state anterior to himself."[24] Freud himself definitively referred to his two dogs as "additions to the family." Animals, then, for both Sade and Freud, ostensibly present aberrations to their dismissive perspectives on Christian love as an unnatural artifice of human civilization—they are exceptions to the limits of neighborliness: Sade, who refuses to recognize the other-as-neighbor (instead submitting them to his will as a non-neighbor), has affection for a dog; Freud—who asserts that one cannot 'love thy neighbor as thyself' (and deploys the outlier of insects to assert the absurdity of universal love), not because they are not a neighbor in the ethical sense (Freud, here, is not appealing to a impulse that would subject all-who-are-unlike-I to maltreatment) but because of love's limits—has affection, and even explicit, self-proclaimed familial love, for animals. Sade and Freud undermine their own 'rational' rejection of neighborliness.

The insight here should be clear: though love and ethicality *can* certainly be bounded, guiding who and how we love (particularly when one lacks the immediate intuition of how an-other should be treated), we must also recognize that there is a pre-ethical dimension of love that can be irreconcilable with (one's own) ethicality. An a-rational modality of love which is severed from the ethical domain and issues from the subject unconsciously. If one can have both neighbors-not-recognized-as-such and love for a dog, then an appeal to ethics as a guiding formulation of love cannot supply a totalizing picture of love's function (how can the love for the animal be operating within an ethical network when the very reason for de-neighboring the non-neighbor is through an appeal to their status as non-human?). My point is certainly not to claim that Sade is somehow redeemed through this love—or even to function as a totalizing explanatory mechanism for why this love exists, or if, in all instances, this can even be called love in the authentic sense. It is, rather, a crevice I wish to pass through in order to understand animality in the dimension of love—and is not, at all, to say that ethicality should not play into the relations between animality and humanity (ethicality *must* intervene in these relations—yet, there is something else already at play). Despite Freud and Sade not recognizing animals as neighbors on the ethical or rational plane, they already treat them as neighbors, and on this plane is a mode of love that enacts (in a limited way) the call for universal neighborliness.

The fact that ethics cannot be relied on as a domain to exhaustively define love does not indicate, of course, that ethics should be abandoned—the highest call of ethics, to love another as if they were oneself (or, in its most powerful crystallization presented by Buddhism: to vacate the content of oneself, and the attachment to that content, for the good of an-other), should not be dispelled simply because of its inability to provide a comprehensive, definitive framework for love—instead, that ethical injunction must be pursued (unless, like Freud and Sade, one pessimistically views it as a theoretical-theological invention that is totally impossible—which I think we must resist), but love must find new grounds (albeit not entirely unrelated to ethical questions), to furnish its explication in the domain of animality. Love for the animal is not merely informed by rational ethical claims.

A Psychoanalytic Account of Love: An Exchange of Lacks

In Plato's *Symposium*, during the meta-dialogue between the prophetess Diotima and Socrates, love is elegantly and almost simplistically defined as "the desire to have the good forever."[25] Subsequently, Diotima articulates love's function: "Love's function is giving birth in beauty in both body and in mind"[26]—and further goes on to explain that, since humans are barred from immortality, they seek to propagate themselves through actual pregnancy, because "reproduction is the closest mortals can come to being permanently alive and immortal."[27] Notably, Diotima explicitly connects this modality of love to animality, stating that "Even the weakest of animals are ready to fight with the strongest and die for their young . . . . The point made about humans applies to animals; moral nature does all that it can to live forever and to be immortal."[28] Pregnancy, of course, does not exhaust this function of love-as-reproduction (as it applies to the human), since there are other, more abstract and non-literal, means of reproduction as well—such as honor, wisdom, artistic production—which all seek to reach "immortal fame for eternity."[29] A few pages later, however, Diotima reveals the absolute highest level of love to Socrates, the recognition of ultimate beauty:

> First, this beauty always *is*, and doesn't come into being or cease; it doesn't increase or diminish. Second, it's not beautiful in one respect but ugly in another, or beautiful at one time but not at another, or beautiful in relation to this but ugly in relation to that . . . . Nor will beauty appear to him in the form of a face or hands . . . or piece of knowledge . . . or as being anywhere in something else . . . . It will appear as in itself and by itself, always single in form.[30]

Progressively, Diotima succeeds in unfurling the greater abstraction of beauty and love until it reaches its ultimate Platonic form in Beauty—an unalterable, atemporal, immaterial modality of beauty that is precisely what the human being seeks: Eternity.

As Diotima clearly elucidates, this abstraction of beauty does not disclose itself to animals—albeit they pursue immortality via reproduction, they do not "understand the reason for it,"[31] unlike humans who can reflect on this pursuit. According to Diotima's schema, animals are left behind in this higher-level love—love as its greatest abstraction in the form of beauty (which, notably, is imbued with the order of the signifier's fabric, as an abstraction voided of reality's materiality)—and animals are left with a corporeal (imaginary), non-knowledge of love-as-love, which would require access to the network of the signifier. Here, we can detect a salient truth revealed by Diotima's discourse with Socrates: Love, when estranged from physicality and the other-as-presence, is unintelligible to an animal. The precondition for animal love is recognition of another in their actual corporeal condition; animal love, always and definitionally, denotes the apprehension of another. There is no such thing as love-of-love for the animal—no idealized, abstracted, incorporeal,

Platonic version of love exists in the domain of animality. (The human condition of romanticizing love is incontrovertibly absent for animals.) Even if one contests Diotima's disquisition on love, on the pretense of clarity or whatever else, the import of the insight on the severance between animal and human love remains. Despite a non-relation to the concept of love as an abstraction in the Platonic realm, animals are clearly situated in the space of relation-to-another, precisely where the entire realm of human-animal relations is positioned.

Lacan devises a formula of love in his seminar on *Transference* as "giving what you do not have,"[32] then he later re-formulates love as giving "what one does not have to someone who does not want it"[33]—which means that one gives their lack, the lack of precisely what they "do not have," to one who cannot bear it or fill it in—the one who is the recipient of this lack (the one who is loved) is not (or *should* not be, since the task is structurally impossible) expected to somehow forever satisfy this lack, to replace it with a jouissance of phantasmic unobtainable non-lack fullness; the loved one is, rather, expected to manage this lack, to assimilate what the lover does not have, in all its delicate, glass-like fragile shatterability, and to, in return, love and care for this lack. The tender exchanges of a loving relationship illustrate this exact dynamic: While one may, publicly, display their achievements and most charismatic, genial, and generally likeable attributes, privately (among those they love), they are relieved of that which makes them lovable to the outside 'audience,' and are free to display lack—their anxieties, fears, insecurities, and those otherwise privatized spheres of self that cannot be, one feels, entrusted to the public. One tells those closest to them (who they love): *Look at my failure; look at that which I cannot achieve; look at that which I cannot be; look at my lack.*

Think about the development of a burgeoning romance—two partners grow closer not by detailing their career successes or agreeable charitability or aspirations (these exchanges are merely the initial stage of becoming acquainted), but through the expression of their failures, of that which they found insurmountable, moments disclosing disagreeable failings, and articulating their laziness and inability to achieve. The same formula for love and lack applies to the triangulation of partners that functions as a trope in romance movies: One woman is split between two (normally radically disparate) lovers, and the viewer has no idea who she really loves, until the precise moment when something tragic occurs—some traumatic incident that she is unable to cope with and must symbolically designate by telling an-other—then we (the viewer) know who she loves by which of the two she tells of this event, and our presumption is further confirmed by their response, by what the recipient does with this lack. The way the other handles this (usually painful) lack is indicative of love.

We desire everyone to perceive our triumphs and recognize that-which-we-have-and-are (our necessarily partial fullness under the guise of a total fullness); we desire those we love to see and love our lack and that which-we-cannot-have-and-are-not. When we give 'what we do not have' to a loved one, we give them access to the emptiness central to our desire—the metonymy of our desire is displayed, without a complete, totalizing object to somehow satiate it interminably.

Desire adheres to an endless deferral prompted by a lack-void; Lacan writes "desire *is* a metonymy,"[34] meaning desire follows the metonymic structure of substitution without a terminating object. In another sense, then, we give the loved one not only what we do not have in terms of what we cannot be or have in ourselves, but also in terms of what we literally cannot *give*—albeit we can love someone, even love them for the duration of our lives, our desire will never be 'resolved' or find a localizable, terminable site in the loved-other to forever occupy in a sustained, immobilized state of satisfaction and content-ness: Our desire is, necessarily, incomplete and evasive, erupting from an ontological lack, and the other will never function as a molar-object to fill in this lack. If we were lackless, of course, desire would not emerge. The memorable (and irrepressibly catchy) line from the 2010s hit "Call Me Maybe" captures this precise meaning of lack: "Before you came into my life, I missed you so bad."[35] We can only make sense of this lyric by reference to lack—one can be "missed" before they even "came into" someone's life because lacking is a state of perpetual missing-ness. In short, the condition of 'missing' (lack) precedes the chance encounter with the loved other because it is concomitant with desire (and love) itself—a subject can miss an object of love before they have knowledge of their existence due to the inherent state of lack that the subject finds themself in. The subject is always 'missing' something (a fundamental lack that submits to the deferral of desire's metonymy), and this is why the encounter with a loved-object appears as a discovery of something that was retroactively missed. Yet, to be psychoanalytically precise, we must slightly modify the formula of the lyrics: *Before you came into my life, I missed you so bad—and after you came into my life, I continue missing, though I offer up my continual missing-ness to you. I will only miss you—even when I 'have' you.*

When we love, we give an-other a modality of desire that we do not possess: A stable, self-sufficient desire that can rest on a single object. This is not to indicate the necessity of polygamy in romantic love (or even the supposedly purely temporal nature of desire and attachment, as something that is subject to gradual attrition)—instead, the object must always be re-configured by the subject in the monogamist relationship, to remain an object of desire, and even with this sustained desire, the object does not 'repair' the subject's lack, with this lack still, of course, haunting a polygamous relationship as well, even one with an endlessly re-iterating successive stream of partners. Lack is not to be 'repaired' because lack is constitutive of the subject.

In the provocative Thailand monologue of the television show *White Lotus*, we see this exact procedure of the limitless deferral of desire: A character, Frank, who has recently become a practicing Buddhist—formerly wildly hedonistic and now celibate and sober—discloses to another character, Rick, the scope of his previous pre-Buddhist exploits, and his realization of their interminable futility. While sipping green tea in a bar, he starts his monologue:

> I moved here because, well, I had to leave the States, but I picked Thailand because I always had a thing for Asian girls, you know? And when I got here,

> oh I was like kid in a candy store. If you've got money, no attachments, nothing to do . . . . I started partying, it got wild. I was picking up girls every night, always different ones; petite ones, chubby ones, older ones, sometimes multiple ladies a night. I was out of control, I became insatiable, and, you know, after about a thousand nights like that, you start to lose it. I started to wonder: Where am I going with this? Why do I feel this need to fuck all these women? What is desire? . . . I realized I could fuck a million women, I'd still never be satisfied—maybe what I really want is to be one of these Asian girls.[36]

Eventually, he pursues a new avenue of pleasure, placing an ad looking for a 'white guy' his age (who resembles him) to have intercourse with, as he 'put[s] on some lingerie and perform[s]' to look like a 'lady boy' from Thailand—inverting his normal position in intercourse and thereby re-configuring himself as the previous object of his desire, the 'Asian girl.' He repeats, again and again and again, this staged sexual positional inversion, confessing that he became 'addicted' to it. After exhausting this, he realizes he was only eluding the true question of desire by 'trying to fuck' his way 'to the answer,' and becomes a Buddhist, rejecting the 'never-ending carousel of lust and suffering.'

Frank's monologue, received by many viewers as utterly cryptic and bizarre, perfectly articulates Lacan's postulation of desire as endlessly deferred and contingent on a constitutive lack: Frank, despite obtaining precisely the object of his desire—in all its iterations (petite, chubby, older)—and even radically re-organizing the sexual situation in order to experience the multiplicity of the matrix that constitutes his desire and its object (all the available facets of his desire—all possible angles of the sexual scenario), the lack motivating his desire remains indissoluble and un-filled. Simply, the lack maintains itself in the subject despite arranging desire in every conceivable configuration to exhaust it. Love, albeit certainly distinct from pure desire, similarly cannot restore wholeness to this lack. The difference between love and desire (insofar as they are divisible) is that in love, one offers their lack to an-other. Accordingly, neither monogamy nor polygamy offer a way of resolving the lack that is fundamental to every human subject (since lack is not to be 'resolved').

To understand the Lacanian aphorism of love ("giving what one does not have to one who does not want it") and its full implications for animal-human love relations, we can again reference Plato's *Symposium*: Famously, a speaker at the dialogic symposium, Aristophanes, defines love as physical unification with another, and to substantiate this conception of love, he appeals to a mythic justification—this myth posits a point in pre-history when all human beings were composed of a unified, inseparable pair-of-one, with two heads, four arms, and four legs. (This myth can be read as an inversion of the *White Lotus* monologue: Whereas Frank tries to gain fullness by engaging in all possible iterations of his love, Aristophanes thinks one gains this lack-less state by finding the one true soulmate.) At this time, according to Aristophanes, all humans were complete—and lack is only introduced by a punishment, enacted by Zeus, that split humans into atomized, incomplete halves, doomed to perpetually seek their complementary half, which would effectively render them, through their unification, into a conjoined, non-split, and utterly complete human fullness. Putting aside the mythic character of this articulation of love, Lacan's formulation of love defies Aristophanes' mythic tale of an irrecoverable totality: For Lacan, there is no possibility of completeness; even if one achieves this supposed unification of two-in-love to arrive at the original One, there is always a gap inherent to their being, which introduces an unavoidable lack on the ontological level—even one's perfect match (in another) is unable to penetrate this lack and suffuse it with a non-lack of being. Lacan's lack is not a missing fullness waiting to be plugged through an idealized fusion of soul mates—it is foundationally, and necessarily, unpluggable; a fissure that forever resists wholeness.

Human Lack and Animal Lacking-of-Lack

However, are animals not ordinarily theorized as having a lack-of-lack? Are they not unable to be the recipient of this lack and to initiate (or complete) the transmission of a meaningful response? In Lacanian thought, love is defined by its position in the triadic structure of Other-desire-lack—love is the substance that coheres this formula, the precise formula that underlies all intersubjective relations. Animals, as we have defined the texture of their interiority so far, do not have the same relation to lack or need—to recall Lacan's succinct formula: "desire is neither the appetite for satisfaction nor the demand for love, but the difference that results from the subtraction of the first from the second, the very phenomenon of their splitting."[37] Animals may be able to demand love in the form of need, but they plainly, unequivocally, have a distinct relation to demand (since human demand 'splits' desire from need through the mediation of the signifier's arbitrary nature). Additionally, animals do not have the same lack as humans; they do not have a castrated mode of being (brought about by the inaugural relation to the symbolic universe). Animals lack the human lack that the signifier brings (they *lack*-lack). Consider, again, (from Chapter 3), the animal relation to the primal horde's parricide; there is no such myth for animals because there is no interiorized Law which intervenes in their actions (though this does not mean that there is no fear of punishment or guilt). The symbolic Law, which introduces lack, does not exist in animality. This animal lack-of-lack must be distinguished from human lack of lack (leading to anxiety): A human's lacking of lack is a void of something which should be present (lacking a lack that should, in a healthy human, be there); an animal's lack-of-lack, is an ontological feature (lacking a lack that is structurally alien to them—paradoxically leading them nearer to completeness). Animals lack-of-lack can only be understood from the perspective of the human and should not be understood as a statement of their supposed inferior status.

Is it not the case that love (in a non-abstract, interpersonal sense) can only occur in a symmetrical exchange of lacks, between two parties equally giving that which they do not have (and is this exchange not predicated on an articulation of lack that implies a linguistic transmission or a set of communicative acts)? An animal, then, would be definitionally excluded as an object of love since they are incapable, according to the formula relied on so far, to dispense 'that which they do not have' to another subject. The problematic, not only of non-reciprocal love (such as unrequited love), but also of differential in the ability to share lack, erupts at the site of human-animal love. Animals cannot participate in human love due to lacking the lack on which the circulation of love subsists.

However, consider the human-baby—the penultimate object of parental love; the baby is an object that the parent, at their ideal best, loves above all and dedicates, in a nearly self-sacrificial manner, their own life. Are babies not lacking *lack* in a similar sense as animals? A baby, although human, has not entered the symbolic universe or post-specular imaginary that introduces Law and activates lack, and consequently is at a stage of development that does not structurally consist of the same ontological lack of desire that an adult human does. Babies do not confront, at the center of their being, a lack that spurs desire—they issue demand (in a non-linguistic manner) for bio-needs that must be met (the need for food and comfort), but do not issue insatiable desires until they enter the system of language. The baby, surely, can be loved; and if the baby can be loved, then the animal can be loved—albeit with a distinct investment (we can, of course, detect a difference in a parent's attachment to their child and animal—despite following similar procedures).

In a different, less linguistically refined manner (meaning it does not exist in the symbolic register), the baby and the animal actually *do* offer lack: They offer lack in their very physical helplessness which are bound to a-linguistic emotional processes. A baby's prematurity and inability to exert independent self-sufficiency force a comparable relation to the domesticated pet's utter dependence on the human subject. They do not *desire*, but they do *demand*. The pet in our home, like the baby, depends on our acts to sustain their life: feeding, administering medicine, and generally maintaining their well-being. In this way, the baby and the pet occupy a similar position: The fundamental inability to reciprocate the highest order of love that is expected of us, and that we necessarily expect from another-like-us (an exchange of lacks) to form a symmetrical relationship. This is precisely why the same language is oftentimes employed with a human-child and a pet. The emergence of designations such as 'fur baby' and 'family animal' circulates due to the recognition of their commonalities in this dimension of lack in the domain of demand. However, one must acknowledge that babies are in a developmental phase, lacking something they will receive, while animal's lack-of-lack is not an incompleteness—animals are complete in their own distinct way (in some ways, more complete than humans, with their fundamental lack). Love is not predicated on the subject's capacity to return love in its exact dimension; love does not need to be matched to be authentic and meaningful—though this does tell us something about the distinction between non-romantic and romantic love (since romantic love seems predicated on a symmetrical exchange of lacks, while other modes of love, such as parent-child, or helping a stranger-as-neighbor can be predicated on an asymmetrical exchange).

In a way, an exchange of lack does occur between the animal and the human: We offer animals our lack in desire, and they offer us their lack in demand—an ontological lack exchanged for a physical lack. Further, the animal lack, although a demand in the domain of physicality, does not mean the animal automatically gives up their lack: Yes, they may accept food from anyone who offers it (adhering to 'instinct'), but that does not mean they give up their lack—their fundamental vulnerability, both physical and even emotional—to anyone. A baby helplessly, indiscriminately offers up their lack—a fully formed, adult animal discerningly gives up their lack. An animal that permits themself to be vulnerable, to be taken care of, offers their lack (in the physical sense of a bio-need) to a human. Should we be concerned with reducing the animal (or the baby) to an object, denying them genuine recognition as subjects-of-experience and thereby permitting us to treat them however we'd like in a perverse Sadean manner? No—the fact that love may have an origin other than ethicality as the site from which it erupts does not mean that love disobeys the field of ethics. To truly love the baby, or the animal (going beyond Sade's mere 'affection'), is to treat the baby or animal ethically—though the love in the first place may have an origin outside the ethical dimension. The subject does not (always) love the baby or animal out of an ethical duty—though their love will bind them to ethical acts. (Love does not emerge from logical-ethical syllogisms.) Additionally, this is not done in a self-reflexive narcissistic manner where the subject love an-other due to the enjoyment one derives from them (since this is not a full account of authentic love): love is when one approaches the other-as-other in all their alterity and meet their bio-needs, wants, and demands. Here we see the limits of narcissistic love of the other-as-self.

How, though, do we give an animal our lack? They certainly cannot attend to this lack, in terms of what we'd want from another human—but we still do offer up our lack to animals. Consider the common domestic scene (comparable to the lack-sharing by which we defined love between humans): A person experiences some event—the death of a loved one, a traumatic incident, being fired, or are having a bout of melancholia un-attached to a specified event—and who do they inform of these event and its effects? Who do they disclose this event to and cry to? If one loves an animal, then they could tell the animal as if they were a human loved one—they come home and weep to their pet, offering up their lack. Yes, the animal does not assimilate, on the linguistic level, the meaning of the event, but they act as a recipient of this lack nonetheless (the entire field of animals in therapy is contingent on the veridicality of lack-sharing). To say here that the animal is only to be treated as an object—as a non-subject—would be untrue: the animal is treated as the *subject that they are* on the level in which *they can be recipients of lack.* We can give animals our lack, and they can give us back theirs in another dimension. Perhaps this is why human-animal love appears even more durable than human-human love: Human-human love is predicated on the difficult prospect of delicately handling the other's lack; human-animal love, conversely, involves no such prospect and consequently no possibility of shattering our expectations of lack-handling, of loving the very things we find contemptible in ourselves: once we love an animal, we may love them forever—with no real possibility of heartbreak and irreconcilable arguments and divorce, until mortality introduces itself and true loss enters the scene of love in the form of death. With an animal, unless they somehow truly betray us (if an animal can be said to betray), we take the vows of love seriously: We love them onto death.

Love for an animal, like all love, can be theorized in the negative: It is not, *I love you because of X, Y, or Z*, but rather, *I love you despite the very presence of X, Y, or Z—all of which I loath in another, but love in you!* Love, approached in this way, is more enigmatic and less self-evidently translucent: It is not a transactional exchange of *attributes I enjoy* which equals *the person I love* but instead *attributes I do not enjoy* which equals the *person I must love because I am compelled to love them by some non-factor.* Love becomes an a-rational configuration of desire that is independent of what one *wants in another* (there are, of course, limitations to this). This same operation, of love's a-rational, non-relation to desired attributes and characteristics of another, is at play in Marcel Proust's novel, *Remembrance of Things Past*, when Swann, a man of refined taste and high social status, falls in love with a woman named Odette:

> [H]e tried at least to ensure that she should be happy in his company, tried not to counteract those vulgar ideas, that bad taste which she displayed on every possible occasion, and which in fact he loved, as he could not help loving everything that came from her, which enchanted him even, for were they not so many characteristic features by virtue of which the essence of this woman revealed itself to him?[38]

Swann would not say, *I love Odette because of her tastes*, but rather, *because I love Odette, I love her "vulgar" tastes*. He is compelled to love these tastes, not because he agrees with them or even likes them, but *out of his love for her that transcends any given attribute*—the tastes reveal her "essence," and it is this which he loves. Swann's love for Odette imbues all of her with a love that emanates from her being, descending to even the 'bad,' 'vulgar' attributes that are constitutive of an-other.

One should not misapprehend this as a sort of love-calculus where what one loves overpowers what one does not love about another: It is, instead, the case that love irrationally covers the entire scene that constitutes an-other—inflecting even the most 'hated' elements in a hue of love. This is precisely why love is commonly characterized as an irrational gesture of emotion. Swann's love functions in this exact register, showing love not as emanating from definable and localizable characteristics, but instead, more mysteriously, love issuing from an-Other place (the Other of the unconscious). In the case of Swann, his love for Odette explicitly does not emerge from her attributes, such as physical beauty; instead, he realizes his love for her when he recognizes her similarity to a painting. When he realizes the similarity between Odette and "the Zipporah" of an artist named Alessandro de Mariano, she becomes, for Swann, "an inestimably precious work of art"[39] and everything about her is irrevocably suffused with love (though this love gets complicated later in the novel).

It is crucial to observe that this love is not mere fantasy: The undesirable characteristics of another are not elided, thereby generating a fantasy-of-the-other that negates the actual other in their alterity; instead, those characteristics are contended with and *loved*—the peculiar, individuated alterity of the other is loved. Authentic love confronts the Otherness of the other. Bruce Fink explains in his book *Lacan on Love* that the Lacanian formulation of love "must involve a two that remains two—a two that does not collapse the Other into the One."[40] Again, this places Lacan in opposition to Aristophanes and his notion of love as a communion of One: The unification of love (to produce the One) deducts the Other of their alterity, and this very alterity is necessary to the formation of authentic love. In love, the specificity of the Other cannot be negated (love without the alterity of the Other is merely love of oneself). Again, to be emphatic on this point: the loved one cannot be negated; to love, one must contend with the otherness-of-the-other—and on this level we must take their singular lack into account. To love an animal, they must be recognized as beyond-objects—as irreducible and singular subjects with their own wants, demands, and needs.

The human love for animals follows these two formulae established so far: While it is true that when we love an animal, we love someone that is lacking-lack and cannot assimilate the notion of that-which-we-do-not-have, it is also true that we nonetheless offer them our lack, and we love them despite the attributes that we may, otherwise, find contemptible. In short, to convert this into two Lacanian aphorisms: *We give animals what we cannot give*, and *we love animals for what they do not have.* We love animals because we share our lack with them (which they offer back, albeit in a different register), and this love, issued from the unconscious, suffuses their entire being (regardless of the total-whole of their, potentially vulgar or annoying, particularities). The enigmatic nature of love, and its resistance to pure tabulation (the like/dislike calculus), is due to love's orginary source: the domain of the Other of the unconscious. Fink maintains that "the unconscious is always at work in love."[41] We do not simply choose to love—and we do not always (consciously) choose who we love—which is precisely why animals can occupy a position as objects of our love. As should be transparent by this juncture, the psychoanalytic situation of animal-human love cannot collapse into human-animal love (or even animal-animal love, which presents us with its own mysteries). This is precisely why romantic love with an animal, by a human, is a perverse, universally contemptible gesture: The asymmetrical dimension of lack and the utter impossibility of their legitimate exchange totally forecloses that as an authentic option. Romantic love, by a human, is founded on the returned demand for the other's lack in the same domain of desire, which an animal cannot return.

The unconscious origins of love disclose why human-animal love was a coherent possibility for those figures who (in my view, wrongly) rejected the Christian commandment of universal ethical love and neighborliness—Freud, who dismissed the commandment on psychoanalytic grounds of a distinct, exhaustible ethics of drives and the libido; Sade, who denied the commandment on very different grounds of 'rational' anti-ethicality. This does not exhaust love's emergence—since it can unequivocally be derived from ethical judgments as well (loving an-other out of an ethical duty, for instance). Instead, it informs us why a mode of love and care exists even for those who deny loving the animal-neighbor. The question of what is to be done with this lack is an entirely other domain, which is the precise dimension of ethicality (how one is to orient their love is determined by the ethical field). Recognizing this is not a denial of the field of ethicality, but rather an affirmation that, regardless of the progress of ethics in its theoretical or material iterations, human-animal love (recognition of the animal-as-neighbor) is not only a possibility but is already, in fact, enacted. Humans love the animal not only because they *must* but also because they *do*.

Notes

1 Sigmund Freud, *Civilization and Its Discontents*, trans. James Strachey (New York: W. W. Norton & Company, 1961), 65–66.
2 Proust, Marcel, *Within a Budding Grove*, trans. C. K Scott Moncrieff and Terence Kilmartin (Modern Library New York, 2003), 154.
3 Marquis de Sade, *Justine, or The Misfortunes of Virtue*, trans. John Phillips (Oxford: Oxford University Press, 2006), 142.
4 Sade, *Justine*, 142.
5 Freud, *Civilization and Its Discontents*, 66–67.
6 Jacques Lacan, *The Ethics of Psychoanalysis: The Seminar of Jacques Lacan, Book VII*, ed. Jacques-Alain Miller, trans. Dennis Porter (New York: W. W. Norton & Company, 1992), 186.
7 Lacan, *Ethics of Psychoanalysis*, 193.
8 Jacques Lacan, *Anxiety: The Seminar of Jacques Lacan, Book X*, trans. A. R. Price (Cambridge: Polity Press, 2014), 26.
9 Bhikkhu Bodhi, ed., *In the Buddha's Words: An Anthology of Discourses from the Pāli Canon* (Boston: Wisdom Publications, 2005), 348.
10 Teddy Duncan, Jr., *Interpreting Meat: Theorizing the Commodification and Consumption of Animals* (Jefferson, NC: McFarland, 2024), 176.
11 Duncan, *Interpreting Meat*, 176
12 Slavoj Žižek, "Kant and Sade: The Ideal Couple," *lacanian ink* 13 (1998): 12–25.
13 Jacques Lacan, *Écrits*, trans. Bruce Fink (New York: W. W. Norton & Company, 2006), 648.
14 Lacan, *Écrits*, 659.
15 Lacan, *Écrits*, 659.
16 Lacan, *Écrits*, 659.
17 Lacan, *Écrits*, 660.
18 Lacan, *Ethics of Psychoanalysis*, 189.
19 Lacan, *Écrits*, 667.
20 Lacan, *Écrits*, 656.
21 Lacan, *Écrits*, 667.
22 Jelica Šumič, "Is There a Politics in Psychoanalysis?" *Política Común* 9 (2016).
23 Roland Barthes, *Sade, Fourier, Loyola* (Paris: Éditions du Seuil, 1971).
24 Élisabeth Roudinesco, *Freud: In His Time and Ours*, trans. Catherine Porter (Cambridge, MA: Harvard University Press, 2016), 242.

25 Plato, *The Symposium*, trans. Christopher Gill (London: Penguin Classics, 1999), 43.
26 Plato, *The Symposium*, 43.
27 Plato, *The Symposium*, 44.
28 Plato, *The Symposium*, 45.
29 Plato, *The Symposium*, 46.
30 Plato, *The Symposium*, 49.
31 Plato, *The Symposium*, 44.
32 Jacques Lacan, *Transference: The Seminar of Jacques Lacan, Book VIII (1960–1961)*, ed. Jacques-Alain Miller, trans. Bruce Fink (Cambridge: Polity Press, 2015), 129.
33 Jacques Lacan, *Crucial Problems for Psychoanalysis: The Seminar of Jacques Lacan, Book XII (1964–1965)*, trans. Cormac Gallagher, unpublished translation from unedited French manuscripts, accessed via lacaninireland.com, 165.
34 Lacan, *Écrits*, 439.
35 Carly Rae Jepsen, "Call Me Maybe," by Carly Rae Jepsen, Josh Ramsay, and Tavish Crowe, recorded 2011, track 1 on Curiosity, 604 Records/Schoolboy/Interscope, 2012.
36 Mike White, creator, The White Lotus, season 1, HBO, 2021.
37 Lacan, *Écrits*, 580.
38 Marcel Proust, *Remembrance of Things Past*, vol. 1, trans. C. K. Scott Moncrieff and Terence Kilmartin (New York: Vintage Books, 1982), 268.
39 Proust, *Remembrance of Things Past*, 245.
40 Bruce Fink, *Lacan on Love: An Exploration of Lacan's Seminar VIII, Transference* (Cambridge: Polity Press, 2016), 103.
41 Fink, *Lacan on Love*, 120.

Conclusion

The Ethics of (Zoological) Psychoanalysis

The most compelling questions to those in the humanities and social sciences are precisely those which I do not contend with in this book, namely, the questions seeking to move towards resolving ethical 'real-world' problems. I am not, in any way, indifferent to the ethical treatment of animals or their moral status (as I've said elsewhere, we must love the animals other as *other* and this mode of love certainly comes with ethical obligations), yet this book is not about the ethical status of animals. To be impossibly clear: The psychoanalytic insights I arrive at are not prefigured to ratify an ethical stance towards animality—the concepts I develop are the result of analyzing the terrain of animal interiority in the psychoanalytic register, and all ethical implications are mainly secondary (though I do contend with them in Chapter 5). The ethical questions can only be asked once the interiority of animals has been elucidated—and this book only offers the initial elucidation.

Ethics is certainly a precarious topic for Lacan due to the intervention of the unconscious in one's (conscious) intentionality. As he writes in Seminar V: "fiction aside, there is really no more common experience than that not only are our reasons for doing things incoherent, but we don't know what those reasons are and are fundamentally alienated from them."[1] Our reasons for action—whether ethical or not—do not emerge from perfectly rational reflection; action frequently erupts from the site of the unconscious in a winding, convoluted path that is difficult if not impossible to trace. Our reasons for doing things are fundamentally "incoherent." Lacan certainly does not disavow the ethical field as having no utility—but understanding the subject (and what is beyond the subject, the subject-beyond-subject) can be, at times, discordant with ethics. Understanding a subject (what they *are*) and understanding ethics (what one *should do*) are two distinct inquiries—for animality (a subject where how one should act has no bearing on ontological or phenomenological understanding—meaning animal being is being regardless of the ethical field, not taking into account, of course, the individuated animal experience which is directed by ethical, or unethical, action on behalf of humans) asking ethical questions is directed towards the human, leaving the animal outside one's scope.

Towards the end of Lacan's seminar on *The Ethics of Psychoanalysis*, he leaves the reader with a well-known, ambiguous aphorism on ethics: "The only thing one

DOI: 10.4324/9781003635383-9

can be guilty is of having given ground relative to one's desire."[2] What does Lacan mean by this opaque statement, putatively resolving fundamental questions around desire, guilt, and ethics? He means guilt comes not (only) from the (occasionally) opposing poles of desire and good, but also from negating one's desire in the name of good (or even the social 'good' that defies the ethical good), denying one's own desire to correspond with the social Other's demands. One can be guilty not only of acting out one's desire against good, but of severing off one's desire—acting as if it did not exist (or perhaps actually being unaware it exists)—due to the social imposition of the good or 'false-good' upon one's desire. I re-articulate this aphorism, for my purposes, to read: *The only thing the theoretician can be guilty of is having given ground relative to theoretical truth.* Truth, like the truth-of-desire (not the fact of acting in accordance with desire but recognizing its existence), can never be in contention with ethicality: The ethical arena can withstand anything emerging from the domain of truth. If I conclude that the animal has access to the sign but not the signifier—communication but not language—this does not in any way attenuate the moral considerability of animals. Similarly, the contention that animals have subjectivity (specifically, a subjectivity structured by the imaginary field) and an unconscious exceeding instinctual activity is not asserted for ethical reasons (though it may have ethical implications). The fact that animals deserve ethical consideration—to be treated as subjects in all their alterity—is not contingent on their status as psychoanalytic subjects and the structure of their interiority.

Academics studying animal consciousness and being who insist on the ethical power or pragmatic, 'real-world,' utility of their scholarly contributions risk potentially engaging in a backwards procedure: Starting from an ethical value to derive a theoretical (or even worse, faux-empirical) truth—and this post-hoc sequence, at its best, omits material that is inconvenient and at its worse purposively siphons in, like an ethical vortex acting in the negative, 'truth' to align with a set of (normally socially-sanctioned) ethical presuppositions. In this proclivity there is a crypto-pragmaticism at play, asserting that knowledge's only function is its immediate utility for social optimization. Jean-François Lyotard identifies precisely this as the condition of post-modernity: "Knowledge ceases to be an end in itself, it loses its 'use-value.'"[3] Knowledge is used only to serve "the best performativity of the social system"[4]—and what is ethics if not an attempt to maximize the functioning of a social system towards certain ends? "Performativity" does not only serve capital-accumulation.

My insight here, when I reference theoretical 'truth.' is not to claim I've achieved the "God" perspective of absolute objectivity that Donna Haraway forecloses as a conceivable authorial positionality, calling it "the god trick of seeing everything from nowhere."[5] Haraway deftly articulates that objectivity in this sense is an utter impossibility that only functions to conceal its partiality. Haraway, in her book, *Simians, Cyborgs and Women*, conversely calls for "situated knowledges"—what she designates "feminist objectivity"—a view that acknowledges its own partiality and the impossibility of a totalizing, "unmarked"[6] perspective.

I undeniably must concede that *Zoological Lacan* has, like any other text, a marked perspective—my writing is refracted through all the texts referenced and influenced by my own subjectivity. I do not, though, take the next step that Haraway declares necessary—where a given subject-position is submitted to interpretation (meaning one's 'interpretation' is subject to an interpretative—ethical—criteria outside itself), and this interpretation is, for Haraway, bound to a "moral and political discourse" that "should be the paradigm for rational discourse."[7] My analysis takes place within the initial interpretation—subsequent theorists can, if they like, submit it to the secondary ethical-hermeneutical discourse, but I will not, as I must first establish the theoretical truth of animal subjectivity. Although I am willing to call my analysis an 'interpretation'—explicitly announcing my own self-awareness that it is 'marked'—I do not agree with Haraway that this means I must submit it through a prism of ethicality, marking it even further. Would Haraway deny the fact that some perspectives undergo a more convoluted filtration process, abstracting the analysis an additional layer from their subject and making them more marked than others? My book presents a marked perspective, but I wish it to be as *unmarked* as possible, though it will surely be re-marked by others in the ethical or political dimensions.

I refuse the presupposition that a scholar—in any field—is *compelled* to generate ideas immediately applicable to the social world: My function as author and scholar, at least in this text, is not to *liberate* or *subvert* or *mandate*—it is to *theorize* and *interpret*; in this case, to expand the epistemic limits on animal subjectivity in a new domain, namely the domain of Lacanian psychoanalysis. At times, this may align with the political and socio-theoretical goals of activists or social proponents of animal welfare, and at other times, my findings will be major departures from precisely those goals. This is because my text is not seeking a political-material end but rather is a theoretical-becoming: A theoretical text bound to an end is confined, limited, and already-exhausted. Socrates says that theory is the nearest to the truth, asking his interlocutor: "Does practice ever square with theory? Is it not in the nature of things that, whatever people think, practice should come less close to truth than theory?"[8] Theory is truthful because it does not capitulate to the burden that the activation of a reality ("practice") imposes on it—there is no concern with what is 'possible,' but rather only with what is true.

It does not matter, for example, if Socrates theorized Republic was possible—only that it was truthfully the best conceivable state (according to the standards of Plato's version of Socrates and his dialogic characters). I'm far from saying that theory permits one to say anything without concern for reality (there is a binding procedure that secures theory to reality), but rather that a truthful theory, at least in the field of animality, asserts itself without total fidelity to a praxis. One does not need a psychoanalytic confirmation of animals' relation to the imaginary field and the arena of love to treat them ethically—these are only truths about animal subjectivity and phenomenology. Presenting animal interiority truthfully permits an ethical foundation to be constructed—but these activities must be distinct to approach truth.

I do not, however, totally disclaim any ethical or praxis-oriented undercurrents which may punctuate my own text (again, the text is certainly marked, even in ways I may be unaware of): I personally have an ethical stance towards animals and their real-world treatment, especially apparent in my first book, *Interpreting Meat*, and in my personal activity as a vegetarian. In *Interpreting Meat*, though I explicitly avoid 'prescribing specific legislative or personal action,' the entire project of confronting the human consumption of meat, in the manner I did, is predicated on an implicit, but unequivocal, ethical claim: That there is something about animality which renders the eating of meat symptomatic, forcing it to stick out in human consciousness. Now, in this book, though I certainly approach animality with my own presuppositions, there is no ethical nexus that the text is predicated on—my own (ethical) view of animality is not at stake in theorizing the interiority of animals, though the choice of animals as a subject for the book is certainly latently indicative of my stance on the treatment of animals.

Lacan, in a gesture that repudiated the prevailing psychoanalytic approach of ego-psychology, frequently averted straight-forward normative claims and ethical mandates. The ego-psychologists wanted the analysand to cultivate a 'strong' ego predicated on the analyst's own ego, but the problem is that this rendered the point of analysis for the analysand to identify with the analyst: An analysis designated as 'successful' was wholly dependent on the analysand aligning with the analyst, of structuring their ego according to the analyst's. Despite Lacan distancing himself from the moralizing field of identification with the analyst's own ego-morality—Lacanianism wholly embraces love. Lacan writes, paraphrasing a French politician: "politics is politics, but love always remains love."[9] If politics is the social instantiation of ethics qua Law, then it is susceptible to the binding effect of reality, where ethical possibilities are circumscribed to what is politically viable—what can be done within a certain social epoch restricted by a particular socio-political configuration. Love, conversely, is not subjected to political viability: It is extra-political and even extra-ethical, though never unethical. I think this should clear up why my book revolves around a theory of love rather than the ethical field.

Notes

1 Jacques Lacan, *The Formations of the Unconscious: The Seminar of Jacques Lacan, Book V*, ed. Jacques-Alain Miller, trans. Russell Grigg (Cambridge: Polity Press, 2017), 40.
2 Jacques Lacan, *The Ethics of Psychoanalysis: The Seminar of Jacques Lacan, Book VII*, ed. Jacques-Alain Miller, trans. Dennis Porter (New York: W. W. Norton & Company, 1992), 319.
3 Jean-François Lyotard, *The Postmodern Condition: A Report on Knowledge*, trans. Geoff Bennington and Brian Massumi (Minneapolis: University of Minnesota Press, 1984), 7.
4 Lyotard, *The Postmodern Condition*, 48.
5 Donna J. Haraway, *Simians, Cyborgs, and Women* (London: Free Association Books, 1996), 189
6 Haraway, *Simians, Cyborgs, and Women*, 189.
7 Haraway, *Simians, Cyborgs, and Women*, 194.
8 Plato, *The Republic*, trans. Desmond Lee (Penguin Classics, 1999), 191.
9 Jacques Lacan, *Transference: The Seminar of Jacques Lacan, Book VIII*, ed. Jacques-Alain Miller, trans. Bruce Fink (Cambridge: Polity Press, 2015), 324.

Index

For Product Safety Concerns and Information please contact our EU representative GPSR@taylorandfrancis.com Taylor & Francis Verlag GmbH, Kaufingerstraße 24, 80331 München, Germany

Batch number: 10725966

Printed by Printforce, the Netherlands